Prostate Health Guide

A Doctor's Framework for Lifelong Men's Health and Vitality

By

Dr. Farhan Mehmood

FARHAN MEHMOOD

Copyright © 2025 by Dr. Farhan Mehmood

All rights reserved.

No part of this publication may be reproduced, stored in a retrieval system, or transmitted in any form or by any means—electronic, mechanical, photocopying, recording, or otherwise—without the prior written permission of the publisher, except in the case of brief quotations used in critical articles or reviews.

Publisher: Publishing Hawks

ISBN: 978-1-7642457-3-9

DISCLAIMER

This book is intended for informational and educational purposes only and should not be used as a substitute for professional medical advice, diagnosis, or treatment. Always seek the advice of your physician or other qualified healthcare provider with any questions you may have regarding a medical condition.

The author and publisher disclaim any liability arising directly or indirectly from the use or misuse of the information contained in this book.

All patient names and identifying details have been changed to protect the privacy and confidentiality of individuals. Any resemblance to real persons, living or deceased, is purely coincidental.

FARHAN MEHMOOD

DEDICATION

For the men who asked the hard questions—and the families who stood beside them.

PROSTATE HEALTH GUIDE
TABLE OF CONTENTS

DISCLAIMER 3

DEDICATION 4

INTRODUCTION 1

CHAPTER 1: THE PROSTATE CANCER EPIDEMIC: WHAT 9/10 MEN MISS ... 6

FREE GUIDE: PROSTATE HEALTH STARTER KIT 20

CHAPTER 2: HOW PROSTATE CANCER WORKS 21

CHAPTER 3: NAVIGATING TESTS, BIOPSIES, AND SECOND OPINIONS 35

CHAPTER 4: MEDICAL BREAKTHROUGHS: SURGERY, RADIATION, AND EMERGING THERAPIES 52

CHAPTER 5: THE ANTI-CANCER DIET: 10 FOODS THAT SHRINK TUMORS 69

BONUS GIFT: TOP 7 FOODS FOR A HEALTHY PROSTATE 86

CHAPTER 6: ALTERNATIVE THERAPIES THAT WORK (AND THE SCAMS TO AVOID) 87

CHAPTER 7: THE 90-DAY PROSTATE RESET 108

CHAPTER 8: THE LONGEVITY PROTOCOL 127

CHAPTER 9: THRIVING BEYOND CANCER 144

CONCLUSION: DESIGNING YOUR PROSTATE HEALTH FUTURE 159

THANK YOU FOR READING .... **Error! Bookmark not defined.**

ABOUT THE AUTHOR 161

REFERENCES 162

GLOSSARY OF TERMS 173

INTRODUCTION

"We need a biopsy," Dr. Brown murmured as he scribbled notes.

Jim sat in his doctor's office, gripping the armrests of the chair as if they were his lifelines. At 62, a retired high school teacher with a love for hiking, he had always felt healthy. But his PSA test—a number he barely understood—had climbed to 6.4.

Jim's mind raced. Cancer? Surgery?

"Would I still be myself afterward?"

Driving home through the quiet suburbs, he felt a weight pressing down on him. *"Why is this so hard to figure out?"* he muttered, staring at the road.

That night, Google showed him a dizzying mix of hope and fear: urgent surgery, miracle diets, and horror stories of side effects.

Jim's story isn't unique—it's the story of millions of men facing prostate cancer, lost in a sea of fear and confusion.

Prostate cancer is a silent giant, affecting 1 in 8 men. In 2023 alone, the *American Cancer Society* reported 288,300 new cases in the U.S. alone.[1]

For many, like Jim, it's a shock—because it often develops without symptoms until it becomes impossible to ignore. Yet here's the truth: prostate cancer is one of the most treatable cancers when caught early. Even in later stages, informed decisions can significantly improve your outcome.

The catch? You need a clear path through the maze of tests, treatments, and conflicting advice. That's why I wrote this book.

As a doctor who has spent over five years treating and interacting with cancer patients in hospitals from Pakistan to the United Kingdom, my passion for prostate cancer is deeply personal. It started with my grandfather, whose struggle with the disease showed me how little patients are informed about their options.

I've seen men in rural clinics with no access to specialists and men in state-of-the-art facilities share the same fears: *Will I survive? Will treatment ruin my life?*

And for caregivers—wives, daughters, partners—the questions are just as urgent: *How do I help without falling apart?*

The healthcare system often leaves you with more questions than answers. Doctors often rush through appointments, tossing out terms like *"Gleason score"* or *"active surveillance"* without explaining their meanings. Online searches can be overwhelming, with some sites urging immediate action and others promoting unproven cures. It's no wonder many men feel paralyzed, and caregivers burn out trying to fill the gaps.

This book is built on a simple yet powerful idea: you don't have to choose between blindly trusting doctors and relying on untested remedies. Instead, I'll guide you through the 3-Pillar Protocol, a balanced approach that combines the best of mindset, nutrition, and evidence-based medicine.

You'll learn when surgery or radiation is the right choice and when watchful waiting is a better option. You'll discover seven research-backed foods that can help shrink tumors, along with affordable meal plans to make them a part of your diet. Plus, you'll find strategies to address the shame or fear that often silences men, with guidance on rebuilding intimacy and purpose after a diagnosis.

Whether you're facing aggressive cancer, exploring prevention, or supporting a loved one, this protocol adapts to your needs, not the other way around.

What will you gain from these pages? Clarity, for starters. No more deciphering medical jargon alone. I'll walk you through PSA tests, biopsies, and treatment options using plain language and easy-to-use tools, including flowcharts to help you determine if a biopsy is necessary.

You'll feel empowered to make choices that fit your life, avoiding the regret that haunts 1 in 3 men after treatment. You'll find hope in stories like Tom's, a 55-year-old accountant who avoided surgery through diet and active surveillance, or Sarah's, a wife who learned to support her husband without losing herself. And you'll save money with practical tips, such as choosing affordable, lycopene-rich foods instead of expensive supplements.

Caregivers, you're not forgotten—there's a chapter just for you, filled with tips to stay strong while helping your loved one thrive.

This isn't just a book; it's a toolkit for action. You'll find checklists, such as **"10 Questions to Ask Before a Biopsy,"** to ensure you're never caught off guard. A 7-day anti-cancer meal plan comes with a shopping list to make nutrition easy.

At the end of some chapters, you'll find resources such as the Prostate Health Starter Kit, which includes a PSA tracker and additional resources. These resources turn knowledge into results, whether you're preventing cancer, navigating treatment, or rebuilding your life afterward.

Beyond my years in oncology, I'm driven by a promise to make cancer care clearer and kinder. My grandfather's battle taught me that medicine is more than just prescriptions—it's about empowering people.

My experience in diverse healthcare systems, ranging from resource-scarce villages to state-of-the-art hospitals, provides me with a unique perspective.

As I pursue integrated medicine, I'm committed to combining conventional treatments with holistic strategies, ensuring you get the best of both worlds.

Remember, you're not powerless against prostate cancer!

This book is designed to help you move from fear to confidence. Turn to Chapter 1 to uncover the truths about prostate cancer that most doctors don't share.

PART 1
DECODING PROSTATE CANCER

CHAPTER 1
THE PROSTATE CANCER EPIDEMIC: WHAT 9/10 MEN MISS

"An ounce of prevention is worth a pound of cure."
— ***Benjamin Franklin***

Mike's pulse thumped as he crept down the hall at night, his throat constricting with every step on the cold tile. A faint hum from the air conditioner whispered in his ears.

At 55, Mike was the kind of man you'd envy, a lean marathon runner who logged 30 miles every week. He hadn't seen a doctor in years, and why would he? He felt invincible.

Over the past few months, he'd started waking up many times a night, three or four times, to use the bathroom.

He dismissed it with a shrug, saying, *"Just getting older,"* but his wife, Lisa, wasn't so quick to accept that.

Concern etched on her face, Lisa urged one night, *"You should get that checked."*

"I'm fine, babe," Mike chuckled, waving her off. *"I probably drank too much water."*

Then came a routine blood test, and when he saw the PSA result of 8.2, his heart sank.

The doctor's voice was flat: *"You may have prostate cancer."*

Mike's eyes dropped to the floor as his mind raced: How can this be happening to me?

Mike's story is not unique. It mirrors the reality of hundreds of thousands of men, not because they're careless or weak, but because they were never taught what to look for.

Takeaway:
You don't need to feel sick to be in danger. Many prostate cancers grow silently, showing subtle signs that are easy to ignore until they aren't.

Prostate cancer is the most common cancer among men in Western countries. Since 1990, diagnosis rates have risen by over 30 percent, mainly due to an aging population and better screening.[2] Despite this, more than 34,700 American men still die every year, a number that should be decreasing faster, given today's medical progress.[3]

So, what's the real problem?

It's not that we lack the tools; it's that we lack awareness.

Men like Mike often misinterpret early warning signs, rely on faulty screening tests, and stay silent due to shame or fear.

But silence won't protect you. Knowledge will.

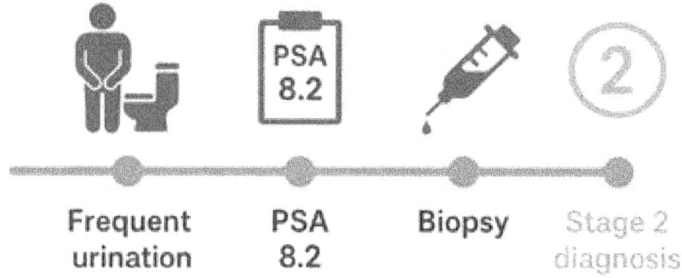

From Early Symptoms to Diagnosis

Frequent urination — PSA 8.2 — Biopsy — Stage 2 diagnosis

In this chapter, you will discover:

- Five early warning signs you should never ignore.

1. Why the PSA test can be misleading and what to do instead.

- How myths of masculinity put men at risk.

- Practical steps you can take, starting today, to stay ahead.

Modern Medicine is Losing the Battle

We live in an age of cutting-edge tools, robotic surgery, advanced imaging, and breakthrough immunotherapies. These aren't science fiction; they save lives in hospitals today.

And yet we're still losing men to prostate cancer.

Here's the paradox:

We're diagnosing more cases but not saving more lives.

According to the *National Cancer Institute*, localized prostate cancer has a 99% survival rate over 5 years. But once it spreads, especially to bones or lymph nodes, that rate drops to just 34%.[4] This drop-off isn't just a number; it's the difference between managing a condition and facing a life-shaking crisis.

The problem? We're not catching it soon enough. And when we do, we often react with the wrong tools.

The PSA Test: More Confusing Than You Think

You walk into the clinic, get your blood drawn, and a few days later, your doctor calls:

"Your PSA is a bit high. We should look into this."

Your stomach drops, but what does that *really* mean?

The PSA (Prostate-Specific Antigen) test measures a protein produced by your prostate. Elevated levels can indicate cancer, but not always.

Here's what the doctors don't always tell you:

2. 40% of men with high PSA don't have cancer at all.[5]
   - Many individuals simply have benign prostatic hyperplasia (BPH) or prostatitis (inflammation).
   - Conversely, 15% of men with "normal" PSA levels do have cancer.[5]

No wonder we get *PSA anxiety.*

One week, you feel fine. And the next you're Googling *"what does a PSA of 6.4 mean"* at 2 a.m., terrified or confused because your doctor didn't explain it well.

A 2021 survey by the *Prostate Cancer Foundation* found that 65% of men felt their doctor didn't explain PSA results clearly. Worse, 20% of men undergo unnecessary biopsies, which can be painful, stressful, and expensive[6]. That's a $1.5 billion burden on the U.S. healthcare system, primarily for tests that didn't need to happen.[7]

Too often, men hear:

"It's just a number. Let's schedule a biopsy."

No context. No nuance. No real understanding.

Key Takeaway:

The PSA test is not a diagnosis; it's a clue.
Knowing its strengths and its flaws can help you avoid panic, over-testing, or missing real danger.

Five Warning Signs You Can't Ignore

Catching prostate cancer early changes everything. Men diagnosed at Stage I have a 99% five-year survival rate. In contrast, those diagnosed at Stage IV only have a 34% survival rate.

This data comes from the *Surveillance, Epidemiology, and End Results (SEER)* program[8]. However, subtle clues can often slip by, sometimes dismissed as signs of aging or hidden by embarrassment.

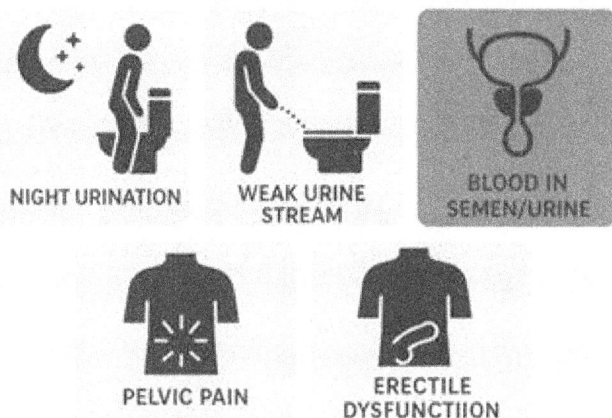

Here are five red flags your body might be signaling right now:

1. Frequent Nighttime Urination (Nocturia)

You wake up once, twice, maybe three times a night to pee. If you're up more than twice, don't brush it off as a regular part of aging. Your prostate rings the urethra like a cuff. When it swells from cancer or a benign growth, it can squeeze your bladder, triggering relentless urges even when it's nearly empty.

2. Weak or Interrupted Urine Stream

You stand... you wait... nothing happens. Then a trickle... then it stops... then it starts again. That stop-start flow often signals prostate pressure on your urethra. Approximately 30% of men over 60 experience this condition, according to the *National Institute of Diabetes and Digestive and Kidney Diseases.*

3. Blood in Your Urine or Semen

You notice a faint pink tinge in the toilet bowl. You blink. *"Did I imagine that?"*

You notice a faint pink tinge in the bowl. You blink. *"Did I imagine that?"* Hematuria (blood in urine) and hematospermia (blood in semen) usually result from infections or minor injuries. But a 2020 study in *Urology* found that in about 3-4% of cases, it's a sign of prostate cancer.[9]

Don't wait for it to happen again.

4. Persistent Back, Hip, or Pelvic Pain

You blame the mattress, your workout, or just the passage of time. But when prostate cancer spreads, it targets bones, especially the lower back and hips. If nagging pain doesn't improve with rest, stretching, or massage, don't assume it's just a result of *wear and tear*. A 2022 study in *Cancer* found that 50-70% of men with advanced prostate cancer reported bone pain.[10]

5. Erectile Dysfunction That Doesn't Make Sense

You take care of your body. You eat well. You exercise regularly. Yet intimacy isn't what it used to be, and it's not just a one-time hiccup.

Erectile dysfunction (ED) can stem from heart issues, stress, or diabetes. However, subtle changes in the prostate can disrupt nerve signals and blood flow long before any other symptoms emerge.

According to the *Journal of Clinical Oncology*, 20-30% of men with undiagnosed prostate cancer report persistent ED.[11]

If you experience new, persistent, and unexplained symptoms, get checked.

Your Body Isn't Betraying You: It's Warning You

These symptoms don't automatically indicate cancer.
They could stem from benign prostatic hyperplasia (BPH), infections, or even stress.

But ignoring them can lead to a late-stage diagnosis and more aggressive treatment.

What to Do Now

- Start tracking your symptoms daily.

3. Schedule a PSA test, but don't rely on it alone; the next chapter explains why.

4. Talk to your partner or a general practitioner if something doesn't feel right.

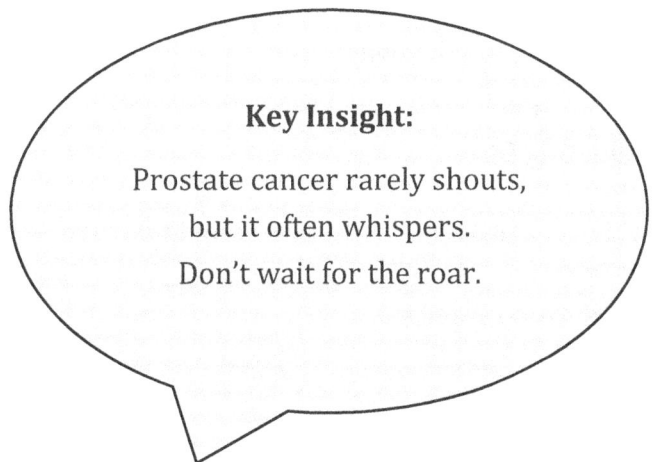

Key Insight:

Prostate cancer rarely shouts,
but it often whispers.
Don't wait for the roar.

FARHAN MEHMOOD
The Toxic Masculinity Trap

Mike wasn't the only one brushing off his symptoms.

In my clinic, I once saw George, a 60-year-old mechanic whose calloused hands smelled faintly of grease. He shifted in his seat, avoiding eye contact as he muttered, *"Doc, I didn't tell my wife... I didn't want her to think I was less of a man."* His voice cracked on the last word.

George had been waking up three times a night to urinate. His stream had weakened, and he had begun timing long drives around bathroom stops. Instead of seeing a doctor, he dismissed it as *"just getting older."* He carried on, silent and stoic, until the PSA results arrived.

We rarely talk about why men like George stay silent.

We're told to:

- Man up.
- Don't complain.
- Don't make a fuss—it's probably nothing.

These aren't just throwaway lines; they become ingrained beliefs that compel men to push through discomfort, downplay pain, and delay care.

But prostate cancer doesn't care how tough you are.

In fact, it thrives on silence.

Why Delaying Isn't a Smart Option

A 2016 study in the *American Journal of Men's Health* found that 35% of men delay seeking medical care for symptoms, compared to just 25% of women.[12] When it comes to prostate issues, the shame runs even deeper. Urination, sexual function, and leakage aren't easy topics to discuss at the dinner table. I've had patients whisper the word "erectile," as if they were confessing something shameful instead of seeking help.

But let me tell you this:

Diagnostic delays significantly increase the risk of advanced prostate cancer.

Often, it isn't the man who notices first; it's his partner asking:

"Why are you getting up so much at night?"

"Didn't you just go to the bathroom five minutes ago?"

"Why are you avoiding intimacy lately?"

These questions are often met with shrugs or jokes. *"I'm just getting old." "Don't worry about it." "I'm fine."*

Behind that casual façade lies a man quietly terrified, unsure of how to express what he is feeling.

Breaking the Trap: Scripts That Open Doors

If you're a man noticing changes, try this statement with a loved one:

"I've been feeling off lately, waking up at night a lot. I think it's time I got it checked. I want to stay strong for us."

If you're a caregiver, wife, daughter, or partner, your words can make a life-saving difference:

"Hey, I read that frequent urination can be more than just aging. Let's get it checked together for peace of mind."

These aren't just words; they're bridges.

They remove the shame associated with symptoms and replace silence with strength.

Because real strength isn't in ignoring warning signs; it's in facing them.

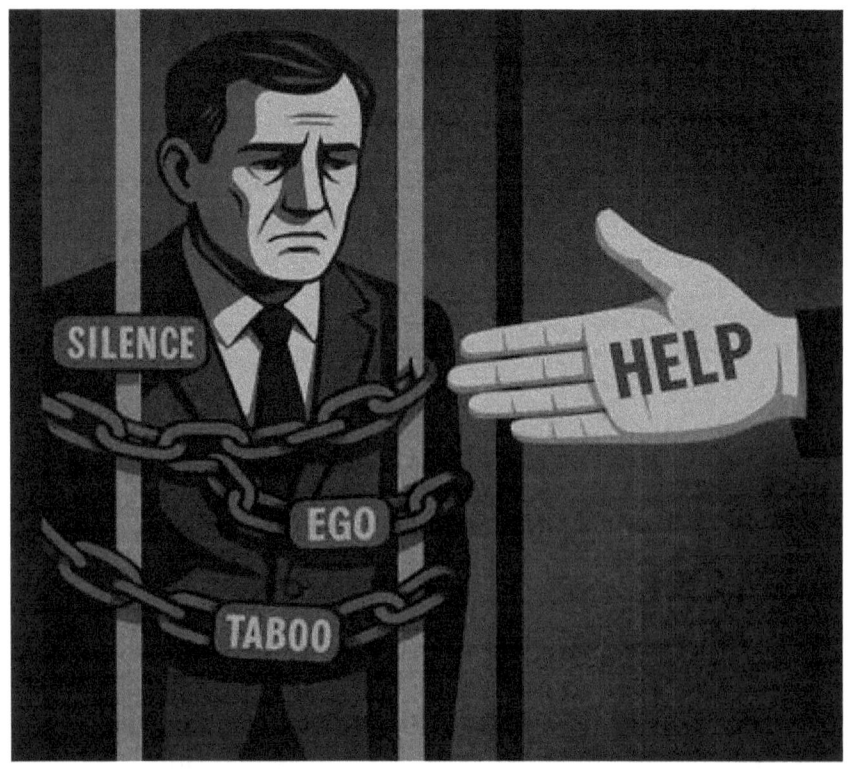

George returned six months after his diagnosis. He was doing well on active surveillance. He looked me in the eye and said, *"I wish I'd spoken up sooner. But I'm glad I finally did."*

Key Takeaway:
Cancer thrives in silence. Speaking up, especially about the uncomfortable stuff, isn't weakness. It's wisdom, courage, and care.

A Marathon Runner's Regret

David never missed a sunrise run. At 48, he was the picture of health, lean, disciplined, and still chasing personal bests in local marathons. When he started waking up at night to urinate and felt a dull ache in his lower back, he shrugged it off.

"Probably just overtraining," he muttered, tightening the laces on his running shoes.

"Maybe take a week off?" his friend Sam suggested. *"I'll be fine. A few extra stretches will fix it,"* David replied, dismissing the concern.

That evening, his wife also nudged him gently.

"You haven't had a checkup in over a year," she said softly over dinner.
"I'm too young for prostate issues; that's for old guys," he laughed. But his body had other plans.

A year passed. The back pain lingered, and nighttime bathroom trips became increasingly frequent. When David finally went for a routine blood test, his hands trembled as he read the results: *PSA 12*. A biopsy confirmed Stage 3 prostate cancer. The news hit him like a punch to the gut.

He underwent surgery followed by radiation. Although he caught cancer before it spread further, the toll was steep. Recovery was grueling, each step a reminder of his body's betrayal.

David struggled with urinary incontinence, something he had never imagined for himself, especially not before turning 50.

He later learned that if he had acted when the symptoms first appeared, he might have qualified for *active surveillance*, a far less invasive approach for low-risk cancers.

Now, David speaks up where he once stayed silent.

"I thought being fit made me safe. I wish I'd acted sooner," he tells other men at support groups.

His story serves as a reminder:

Health isn't just about muscle and mileage; it's about listening to your body when it whispers, not just when it screams.

Facing warning signs head-on transforms fear into power. In Chapter 2, you'll discover precisely how prostate cancer forms and spreads, knowledge that gives you the upper hand.

Key Takeaways

- **PSA isn't a diagnosis—it's a clue.** Understand its limitations before making treatment decisions.

- **Symptoms often whisper, not shout.** Frequent urination, weak stream, or back pain may be early signs.

- **Toxic masculinity delays diagnosis.** Shame and silence are dangerous; speaking up is a strength.

- **Caregivers matter.** Gentle support can prompt life-saving action.

- **Early detection saves lives.** A quick check-up can prevent a life-altering outcome

FARHAN MEHMOOD
FREE GUIDE
PROSTATE HEALTH STARTER KIT

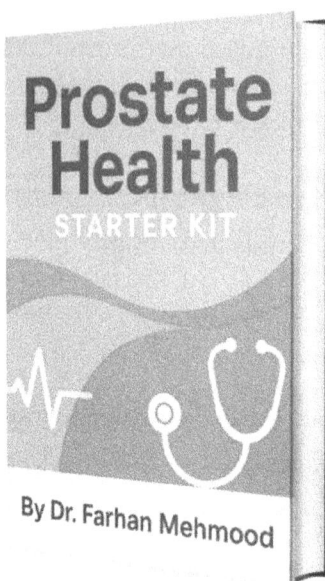

Take control of your prostate health today—**download your free kit (SCAN THE QR CODE ABOVE):**

It includes:

- **Printable 6-Question Self-Assessment**: A quick snapshot of your personal risk.

- **PSA Tracker Chart**: Log your numbers and spot trends over time.

- **Doctor Discussion Guide**: Must-ask questions to bring to your next appointment.

"Should I Get a Biopsy?" Flowchart: A clear, step-by-step decision map.

CHAPTER 2
HOW PROSTATE CANCER WORKS

"Facts are stubborn things, but statistics are pliable."
— *Mark Twain*

Tom, a 60-year-old accountant who lives and breathes numbers, thought he had life all figured out. He jogged daily, ate his greens, and took pride in maintaining his health. But when his biopsy returned *"prostate cancer, Gleason 3+4,"* he felt as if someone had handed him a puzzle in a foreign language.

"What's a Gleason score?" he asked his doctor, who rattled off treatment options like a menu read at lightning speed.

Tom left the office in a daze and later told his daughter, *"It was like listening to Greek."*

That night, shadows danced on his ceiling as he lay awake, his mind racing with questions: What is this cancer doing inside me? Why didn't anyone explain it clearly?

Tom's confusion is all too common. Prostate cancer may be a complex beast, but it doesn't have to be a mystery.

This chapter is your visual guide, breaking down science into clear, empowering snapshots that empower you to face prostate cancer with confidence.

Prostate cancer starts in a small gland tucked below the bladder, a gland that plays a big role in men's health.

Unlike many cancers, prostate cancer often grows slowly; about 70 percent of cases stay confined to the prostate at diagnosis, giving men a high chance of successful treatment.

But it's not always predictable. Some tumors lie dormant for years; others spread quickly to bones or lymph nodes.

Knowing where it starts, how it's graded, what fuels its growth, and what raises your risk is the foundation for smart decisions, whether you're navigating a diagnosis, supporting a loved one, or working to prevent it.

Let's begin by mapping the prostate itself.

The Prostate Map: Where Cancer Begins

Imagine the prostate as a walnut-sized gland nestled below your bladder, wrapping around the urethra, the tube for urine and semen. It's a silent workhorse, producing fluids that nourish and protect sperm. To see where cancer takes root, think of the prostate as a map with four zones.

The *peripheral zone*, located at the back near the rectum, is the largest, about 70 percent of the gland, and it's where most prostate cancers start. The *transition zone*, located closer to the urethra, is smaller but prone to benign prostatic hyperplasia (BPH), a non-cancerous growth common in men over 50; approximately 20 percent of cancers originate here. The *central zone*, around the ejaculatory ducts, and the *anterior zone*, at the front, are rare sites for cancer but can be affected in advanced cases.

> **Did You Know?**
>
> 70% of cancers begin in the peripheral zone.

Understanding these zones reveals why biopsies target specific areas and why a tumor's location can impact your treatment. I once met John, a 65-year-old retiree, who was shocked to learn that his bladder issues stemmed from a transition zone tumor. *"I thought it was just age,"* he said. His biopsy brought clarity and led him to choose active surveillance over surgery.

Like a map, the prostate's zones (as shown in the following diagram) help you chart the course from diagnosis to treatment.

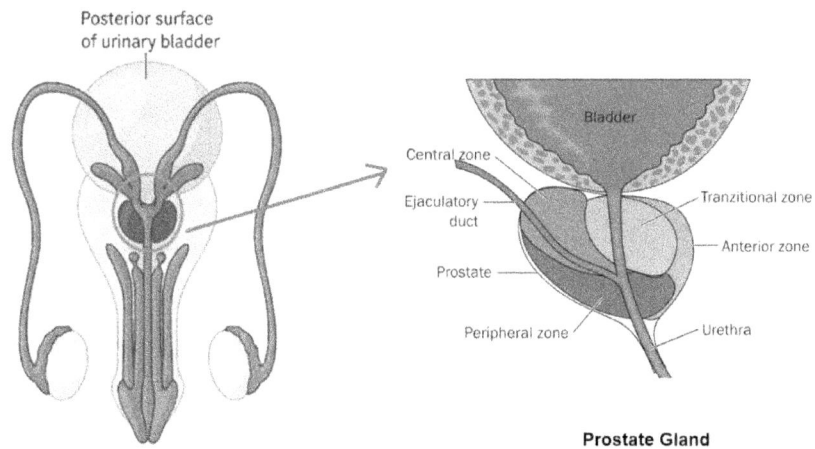

Visual Comparison of Prostate Cells

The following image compares healthy and cancerous prostate cells. On the left, *healthy prostate tissue* shows neat, brick-like glandular structures and uniform nuclei. On the right, *cancerous tissue* reveals disorganized cell growth, enlarged nuclei, and invasive patterns that breach normal boundaries. This side-by-side view brings the table below to life, illustrating the cellular changes you're about to explore.

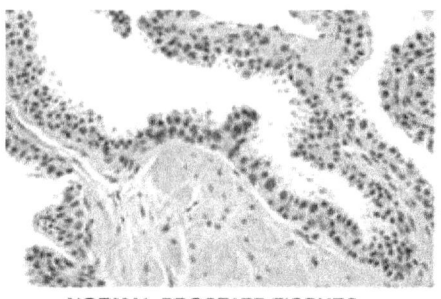 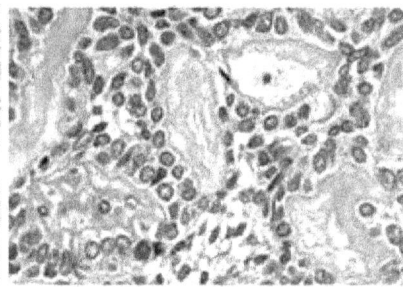

NORMAL PROSTATE TISSUES **CANCEROUS PROSTATE TISSUES**

Feature	Healthy Prostate Tissue	Cancerous Prostate Tissue
Cell Arrangement	Neatly organized, brick-like patterns	Disorganized, chaotic growth
Nuclei (cell center)	Small, round, and regular	Enlarged, abnormally shaped
Growth Pattern	Controlled, cells grow at a normal rate	Uncontrolled, rapid multiplication
Tissue Density	Even distribution of cells and glands	Crowded, invasive structures
Microscopic Appearance	Predictable, well-defined gland structures	Glandular architecture is lost or distorted

Decoding Gleason Scores

What is a Gleason score, and why does it matter?

Your Gleason score is like your cancer's report card. It shows how aggressive your tumor is. Developed in the 1960s by Dr. Donald Gleason, the score ranges from 6 to 10, based on the appearance of the cells under a microscope.

- **Gleason 6** – Low risk: cells look mostly normal.
- **Gleason 3+4** – Mostly slow-growing with some aggressive spots.
- **Gleason 4+3** – Mostly aggressive; higher chance of spread.
- **Gleason 8–10** – High-risk: often needs immediate treatment.

Unfortunately, many doctors don't explain this clearly. That's why Tom was so confused when he heard "Gleason 3+4." It felt like a math problem, not a precise diagnosis. Yet that score can mean surgery or watch-and-wait.

A Gleason score combines two cell grades. Pathologists find the two most common patterns in a biopsy and add them. Each pattern is graded *1* (almost normal) to *5* (chaotic). That is why you see *3+4* or *4+3*. The first number shows the most common pattern, and the second shows the next most common.

Gleason Scores

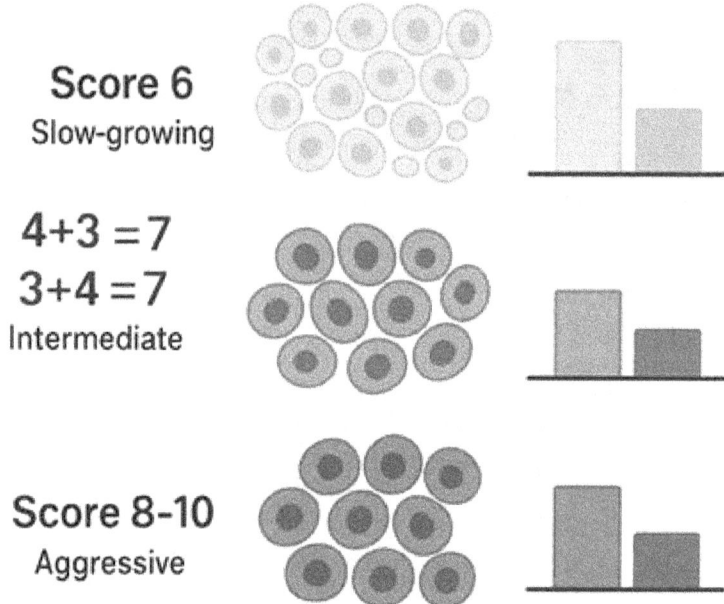

Score 6 — Slow-growing

4+3 = 7
3+4 = 7
Intermediate

Score 8-10 — Aggressive

So, what's the key difference between *3+4* and *4+3*?

Both sum to *7*, but they are not the same. A *3+4* score means most cells are grade *3*—mildly abnormal and slow-growing. A smaller number are grade *4*—more aggressive. A *4+3* flips that meaning, i.e., most cells are grade *4*, making the cancer more likely to grow and spread. That small flip can change your treatment plan.

A *Journal of Clinical Oncology* study found that 60% of men with *Gleason 6* or *3+4* cancer can safely skip surgery and radiation.[13] They choose active surveillance, which includes regular PSA tests, scans, and spot biopsies to monitor for changes. This can spare men from lasting side effects. For example, the *American Urological Association* states that surgery patients have a higher risk of experiencing incontinence or erectile dysfunction.[14] These are not just numbers; they are real lives.

Yet fear often drives overtreatment. A 2010 report in the *European Medical Journal* found that one in three men undergoing prostate surgery had low-risk tumors.[15] Although that figure has declined, it remains far too high.

Sometimes it's due to pressure from doctors; other times it's the emotional weight of a cancer diagnosis. Tom, for instance, was told by his urologist that immediate surgery was the best option for his *3+4 score*. However, after seeking a second opinion, he learned that he was a candidate for active surveillance. With regular monitoring and some lifestyle changes, he could delay or avoid surgery altogether.

For men with higher Gleason scores, *4+3* or *8–10*, cancer is more likely to spread quickly. Research in *Cancer* shows that up to 80% of Gleason *8–10* cases worsen without treatment. That's why prompt action is critical.[16]

Misunderstanding your *Gleason score* can lead to lasting regret. Mark, 58, underwent surgery for a *Gleason 6* tumor, believing fast action was safest until he lived with permanent incontinence. *"If I'd known what a 6 really meant,"* he said, *"I would have waited and watched."*

Your Gleason score is more than a number. It's a roadmap that guides your treatment choices. Knowing and understanding the difference between *3+4* and *4+3* helps you make informed decisions, choose wisely, and protect your quality of life.

The Hormone Connection

Prostate cancer is often seen as a slow-moving disease, but beneath the surface, powerful biological forces are at work, especially hormones.

Testosterone: A Double-Edged Sword

Chief among these is testosterone, the hormone that fuels masculinity. It's key for muscle growth, libido, energy, and overall male vitality. But here's the twist: *while testosterone is essential, it also fuels most prostate cancers.* This double-edged relationship makes managing prostate cancer complex.

Most early-stage prostate cancers are hormone-sensitive, meaning they rely on testosterone binding to androgen receptors to grow. This is why androgen deprivation therapy (ADT) is so effective in these cases.

Androgen Deprivation Therapy (ADT) is a standard treatment for advanced prostate cancer. ADT lowers testosterone to starve the tumor.[17]

ADT Side Effects

ADT delivers strong results initially. It can buy precious time when surgery or radiation alone won't suffice. Yet slashing testosterone comes at a steep price: debilitating fatigue, hot flashes, and bone thinning that can erode your quality of life.

Long-term ADT can cause fatigue, loss of libido, weight gain, hot flashes, and weakened bones. A 2020 report in the *Journal of Frontiers in Oncology* found that nearly 40 percent of men on ADT suffer from bone thinning or loss, raising fracture risk.[18]

Many also report brain fog or persistent low mood. Sometimes it feels like trading one health crisis for another.

It's important to note that *testosterone itself does not cause prostate cancer*. Normal levels are not dangerous. The problem arises when existing cancer cells hijack testosterone to multiply. So, reducing testosterone is about management, not demonization. Balance and personalized care are key.

Stress Hormones: The Hidden Players

Hormones don't stop with testosterone. Stress hormones, primarily *cortisol*, also play a significant role. Chronic stress raises cortisol levels, and high cortisol can harm your health. According to a *Cancer Research* study, chronic stress has been shown to promote the expression of genes linked to tumor growth and metastasis in the prostate.[19] While human evidence remains inconclusive, pathways like immune suppression and hormonal imbalance suggest stress could contribute to prostate cancer progression.

Stress also disrupts sleep, weakens the immune system, and undermines the body's ability to fight illness. I had a patient, Robert, a 62-year-old teacher. During his stressful divorce, his PSA levels spiked. His doctors feared his cancer would worsen. However, after he added daily walks, meditation, and journaling, his PSA levels stabilized without extra treatment. This does not mean stress relief cures cancer, but it is a powerful tool.

Managing Your Hormones

Managing testosterone and cortisol requires more than medication; it calls for changes in your lifestyle, mindset, and daily habits. While doctors may prescribe hormone-blocking drugs, you can control your environment, habits, and stress.

Hormones can either feed cancer or help fight it. Understanding how testosterone and stress affect prostate cancer allows you to make wise, proactive choices. *Balance, not fear, is the key.*

Genetics Risk Factors

Is prostate cancer in your DNA? Sometimes, but genes aren't the whole story. About 10 percent of cases run in families, with mutations like BRCA1 and BRCA2, known for their link to breast cancer, playing a role. According to a study, men with BRCA mutations face a 3.4-times higher risk of aggressive prostate cancer.[20]

James, a 50-year-old patient, discovered his BRCA2 mutation after his brother's diagnosis. *"It was a shock,"* he said, *"but it got me screened early."* If cancer runs in your family, genetic testing can clarify your risk.

Five Lifestyle-Related Prostate Cancer Risk Factors

Most prostate cancers are sporadic, tied to lifestyle and environment rather than genes. Five preventable risk factors stand out:

- **Diet**: While precise figures vary, evidence suggests that diets rich in plant-based foods, especially cruciferous vegetables, help lower prostate cancer risk.
- **Obesity**: Being overweight or obese increases the risk of advanced or fatal prostate cancer by approximately 20–30% compared to men at a healthy weight.[21]

- **Sedentary Behavior**: A sedentary lifestyle can impair immune function and hormone balance, both key factors in cancer progression, even though direct prostate-specific studies are limited.
- **Smoking**: Men with prostate cancer who currently smoke face nearly double the risk of cancer-specific death and about 40% higher risk of recurrence than those who never smoked.[22]
- **Toxins**: Long-term exposure to pesticides has been linked to more aggressive prostate cancer in occupationally exposed groups.

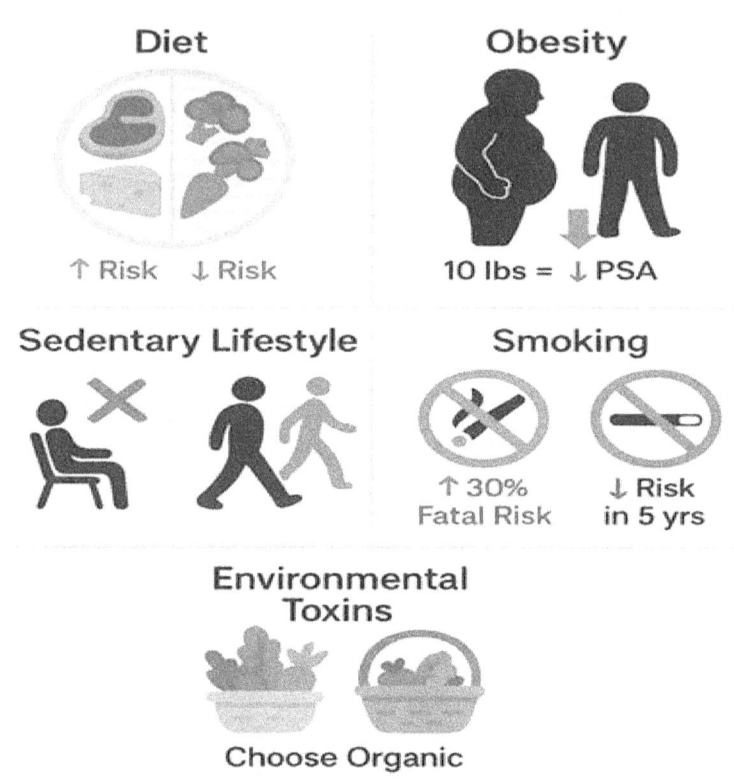

Putting it into Action

After his diagnosis, Tom learned his father had prostate cancer, a clear genetic red flag. He overhauled his life, swapping burgers for salmon, adding daily walks, and quitting smoking. His PSA stabilized, and he avoided surgery. You can't change your genes, but you can tilt the odds in your favor. Caregivers play a role too; encourage a partner to eat more greens or join you on a walk to show support.

Your Next Steps

Genes set the stage, but lifestyle writes the script. Small changes can lower your risk. Understanding prostate cancer, its zones, grades, hormones, and risks transforms your fear into clarity. Tom used his Gleason 3+4 score to choose active surveillance and now hikes with his grandkids. Robert managed stress to stabilize his PSA. James got screened early because he knew his BRCA risk. These men demonstrate what's possible when you understand how cancer works.

In the next chapter, we'll decode diagnosis, PSA tests, biopsies, and second opinions, so you can navigate with confidence. **You're not alone on this journey.**

Key Takeaways

- **Healthy weight matters.** Maintaining a normal weight cuts the risk of advanced/fatal cancer by up to 30%.

- **Move to protect.** Regular physical activity strengthens the immune system and helps balance hormones.

- **Quit smoking.** Halves prostate cancer death risk and lowers recurrence.

- **Eat plants first.** Cruciferous vegetables and plant-rich diets help shield the prostate.

- **Limit toxin exposure.** Reduces the chance of aggressive disease.

- **Combine lifestyle and screening.** Best defense = healthy habits plus timely tests

CHAPTER 3
NAVIGATING TESTS, BIOPSIES, AND SECOND OPINIONS

"The greatest weapon against stress is our ability to choose one thought over another."
— William James

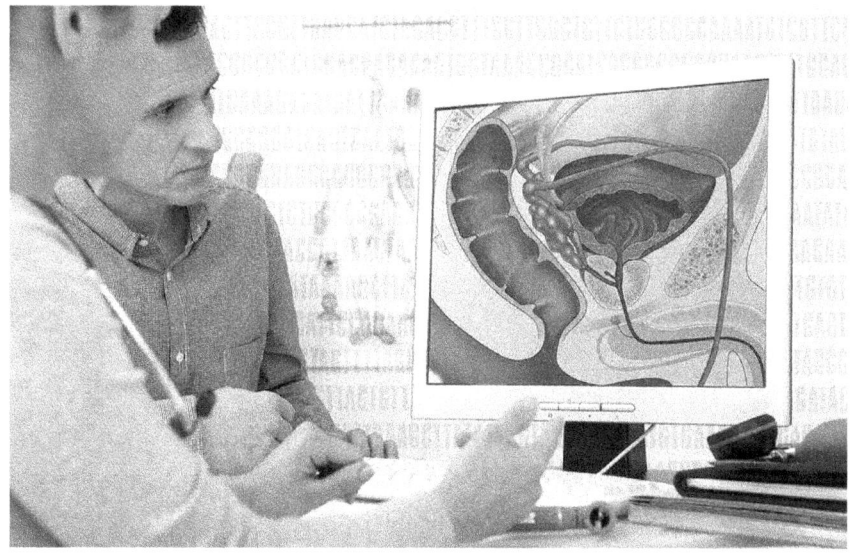

You're at a fork in the road, holding a crumpled map and a single number from your doctor: your PSA. The signposts ahead are faded – one says, *"Prostate Cancer"*, another *"Benign"*, and a third just shrugs, *"Maybe."* Your heart pounds. Is this a life sentence, or a harmless blip? Will your body, your future, your independence be at risk? This is the moment many men find themselves in at the start of a prostate cancer journey: confronted with confusing tests, medical jargon, and urgent choices.

Every year, hundreds of thousands of men face this puzzle. The American Cancer Society estimates more than 313,000 new U.S. cases in 2025.[23] The good news? When caught and managed correctly, the five-year survival rate is close to 98%.[24] Getting the diagnosis right is critical, which means understanding your tests, their limitations, and knowing when to seek a second opinion.

This chapter is your compass through that maze of PSA tests, biopsies, imaging, and second opinions. We'll use real stories and clear explanations to turn confusion into confidence. Think of each section as a landmark on this path – with a metaphorical flashlight to help you see through the fog. By the end, you will have a specific set of steps (an "Actionable Items" checklist) to follow in a calm and controlled way.

PSA Test: Friend or Foe?

James, a 59-year-old accountant, still remembers the day his doctor told him his PSA was 7.2. The number hit him like a freight train. Cancer, surgery, incontinence – all he could picture were worst-case scenarios. Then his urologist calmly asked: "Did you cycle or have sex in the last 48 hours?" The next PSA, taken after James avoided both, fell to 4.1 – back in the safe zone. No biopsy. No panic. In James's case, the PSA test (Prostate-Specific Antigen blood test) was both a friend and a foe: it flagged a problem (good), but it was a false alarm (not cancer).

James's story is a window into the paradox of PSA: it can be a *lifesaving friend* or a *false-alarm foe*.

- **Friend:** PSA can flag prostate cancer early, sometimes before any other test.

- **Foe:** Three out of four elevated PSAs turn out not to be cancer.

- **Confusing:** About 15% of men with prostate cancer still show a "normal" PSA.[25]

So, what exactly is PSA? **Prostate-specific antigen (PSA)** is a protein made by the prostate and measured through a simple blood test. Elevated levels might indicate prostate cancer—but can also signal an enlarged prostate, inflammation, or even everyday activities like sex, cycling, or a rectal exam.

PSA cannot tell you whether a tumor is aggressive or harmless. Its flaws spark what I call "PSA anxiety," that sinking feeling when a single number leaves you fearing the worst. However, once you understand these pitfalls, you can replace fear with clarity and make more informed choices.

Bottom Line:

PSA is a useful clue, not a final verdict. Elevated results don't automatically mean cancer, and "normal" doesn't guarantee safety. Understanding its limits helps you sidestep panic and make smarter choices.

The Four Pitfalls of PSA Testing

James's scare isn't unusual. Here are four ways PSA testing can mislead:

- **False Positives**—most men with an elevated PSA do not actually have cancer. Studies show that nearly 70% of high PSA results don't reflect cancer.[26]

- **False Negatives**—a normal PSA does not guarantee safety. Prostate Cancer Prevention Trials show that around 15% of men with normal PSA still harbor cancer.[27]

- **Everyday Spikes**—activities like cycling, sex, or even a digital rectal exam (DRE) can temporarily boost PSA. For example, in one study, 87% of men saw their PSA rise after sex, and in another, 76% had a PSA increase after a DRE.[28,29] Because of this, doctors often recommend avoiding such activities for 48 hours before testing.

- **No Clue About Aggression**—PSA measures quantity, not quality. A high number may reflect a harmless, slow-growing tumor, while a low number could mask an aggressive cancer.

What Does This Mean for You?

A PSA test isn't a verdict — it's a *clue*, and like any clue, it only makes sense in context.

Consider Carlos's story, which I call *'The Cycling Scare.'* At 58, Carlos was a hardworking chef who loved his morning bike rides. One day, his PSA came back at 6 — a number high enough to make his doctor consider a biopsy. Overnight, Carlos's world turned upside down. He imagined surgery, side effects, and a future he wasn't ready for.

But here's where the story shifts. Instead of rushing into a biopsy, his doctor paused. He suggested a repeat test, this time under controlled conditions: no cycling, no sex, and no strenuous activity for 48 hours. When Carlos went back, his PSA had dropped to 3.8 — well within the safe zone. His "cancer scare" turned out to be an *everyday spike*, caused by lifestyle factors, not disease.

The Lesson?

Never let a single test dictate your future. Always ask for a repeat PSA under controlled conditions before making major decisions. It could save you from unnecessary procedures — and days of needless anxiety.

And that's the bigger picture: *PSA numbers don't live in isolation. They influence your doctor's decisions.* One branch of the flowchart may mean reassurance and watchful waiting. Another may lead to a biopsy, with its own risks and consequences. That's why context, second opinions, and thoughtful decision-making matter just as much as the number itself.

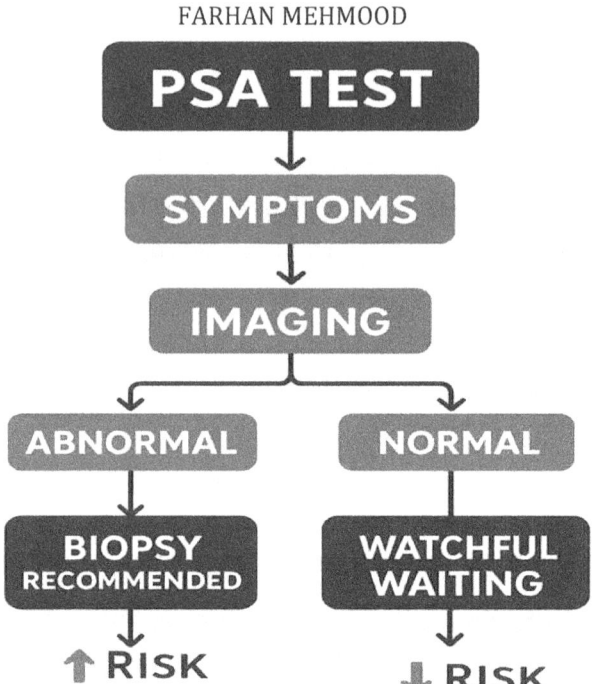

Managing PSA Anxiety

When you're standing at that fork in the road, it's no wonder a single PSA result can send your heart racing. One number might push you toward a biopsy; another might leave you in limbo, waiting for the next test. The truth is, PSA alone is not the whole story — and managing that anxiety starts with *context, not just numbers.*

A smart first step is to repeat the test under controlled conditions. Avoid common triggers — like strenuous exercise or ejaculation — for at least 48 hours before the blood draw. Then, don't just look at the number in isolation; focus on *PSA velocity* — how quickly it's rising over time. In fact, a landmark 2007 *Journal of Urology* study found that the traditional cutoff of 0.75 ng/mL per year missed nearly half of prostate cancers in men under 60. A lower threshold of 0.4 ng/mL per year proved to be more reliable for identifying risk early.[30]

Caregivers also play a powerful role here. If your partner's PSA comes back high, you can be the calm voice in the room. Ask the doctor directly: *"Could this be BPH, prostatitis, or something other than cancer?"* That single question can reframe the conversation and often ease unnecessary panic.

Remember: *a PSA test isn't a verdict — it's a clue.* When you question results, seek context, and look at the bigger picture, you sidestep the anxiety trap and set the stage for smarter, more confident decisions ahead.

Biopsies: Beyond the Pain Myth

When a PSA test raises alarms, the word *biopsy* can feel like a thunderbolt. For many men, it conjures images of unbearable pain and frightening unknowns. But here's the truth: the **myth of the "excruciating biopsy" is far scarier than the reality**. With the right preparation and questions, most men find the procedure surprisingly manageable.

Take Frank, for example. At 62, he was terrified before his biopsy, convinced it would be "the worst pain of his life." His clinic recommended a transperineal biopsy with light sedation. Afterward, he laughed in relief: *"It was easier than my root canal!"* Frank's transformation came not from luck, but from asking questions beforehand that clarified the process and eased his fears. His story proves that fear often comes more from the unknown than from the needle itself.

So, what happens during a biopsy? The most common is the *Transrectal Ultrasound-Guided Biopsy (TRUS)*. A small ultrasound probe is inserted rectally to guide a needle that takes 12–16 tiny tissue samples — the international standard according to the European Association of Urology. Local anesthesia numbs the area, and most men report only mild discomfort.[31]

In fact, the numbers tell a reassuring story. A 2023 *European Urology* study on men undergoing MRI-targeted transperineal biopsies found that 84% reported no or minimal pain, and 80% reported no or minimal discomfort.[32] Severe complications were rare. Minor side effects can happen — blood in the urine (around 18%), blood in the semen (14%), or mild rectal bleeding (about 3%) — but they usually resolve on their own. Infection with fever is uncommon (less than 1%), and severe complications affect fewer than 2% of men, according to *Frontiers in Surgery*.[33]

Even more encouraging: in some cases, a biopsy may not be needed at all. A 2019 *study in Urologic Oncology found that using MRI before biopsy spared nearly 1 in 5 men (19%) from undergoing the procedure without missing any* significant cancers.[34] That's why smart preparation and the right questions can make all the difference.

Think of it this way: walking into a biopsy without preparation is like heading into a storm without an umbrella. Preparation is your best shield. At the end of this chapter, you'll find a **10-point checklist** of must-ask questions, rooted in the 3-Pillar Protocol's call for informed decisions. These questions cut through jargon, clarify your options, and help you step into the procedure with confidence. For caregivers, going through the checklist together answers another key question: *"How can I best support him?"*

Yes, biopsies carry risks. But they are not the ordeal the myths suggest. As Frank discovered, knowledge turned his anxiety into calm. By understanding what's involved, asking pointed questions, and using tools like MRI where appropriate, you sidestep fear and minimize surprises.

Bottom line: A biopsy is a hurdle, not a nightmare. Approach it with preparation and questions, and it becomes a manageable step toward clarity — one that helps you and your loved ones face prostate cancer with strength, calm, and informed choice.

MRI VS. Ultrasound

When a PSA test raises a red flag, imaging is often the next step to sharpen the picture. The question is: which tool should guide you — **ultrasound or MRI**? Think of it like choosing between a flashlight and a spotlight. A flashlight (ultrasound) is inexpensive, handy, and widely available. A spotlight (MRI) is far more powerful, illuminating details that might otherwise remain hidden — but it's harder to access and more expensive.

Important Note:

In this chapter, "MRI" refers to the more advanced multiparametric MRI (mpMRI). Standard MRI alone isn't as effective for prostate cancer detection, while mpMRI more accurately detects aggressive cancers.

For David, a 55-year-old engineer, this difference was life-changing. His PSA was 5.5, and a biopsy seemed inevitable. But his doctor ordered a multiparametric MRI (mpMRI) first. The scan showed no aggressive cancer. David skipped the biopsy and walked away relieved: *"It was worth the hassle,"* he said.

Stories like David's highlight why imaging choices matter. Ultrasound is useful and cost-effective, but its accuracy has limits. mpMRI, on the other hand, detects more aggressive cancers and spares many men unnecessary procedures — but it comes with higher costs and limited availability.

Ultrasound (Flashlight)

- Affordable ($300–$600 on average; a TRUS biopsy runs $1,800–$3,000).[35]
- Widely available in U.S. hospitals.
- Helpful for measuring prostate volume and PSA density.
- **Limitation:** Conventional TRUS can miss up to 25–30% of clinically significant cancers.[36]

mpMRI (Spotlight)

- Excellent at spotting aggressive prostate cancers — catching about 9 out of 10 serious tumors.
- Pre-biopsy MRI allows roughly 1 in 4 men to avoid biopsy altogether.
- **Trade-offs:** Expensive (U.S. average ~$4,400, with some hospitals charging up to $15,000). Not always available. False positives can occur, and approximately 1 in 10 men experience claustrophobia in the tight MRI tube.[37]

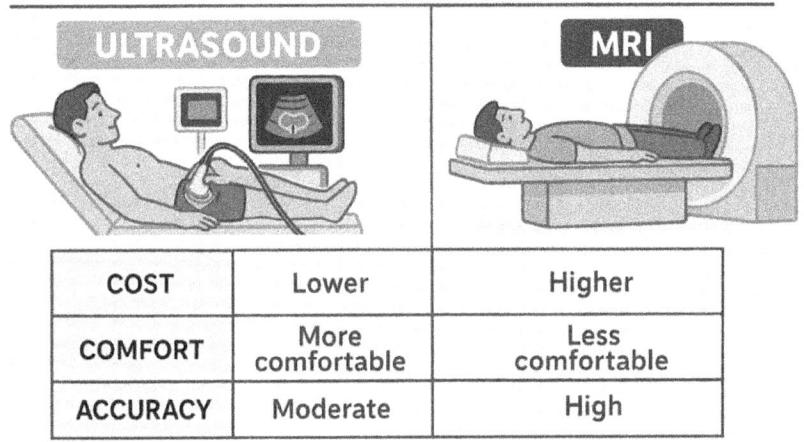

	ULTRASOUND	MRI
COST	Lower	Higher
COMFORT	More comfortable	Less comfortable
ACCURACY	Moderate	High

The bottom line?

MRI shines brighter, but accessibility matters. If you can access it, mpMRI often saves men from unnecessary biopsies and offers clearer insight. If not, ultrasound paired with PSA density still provides valuable guidance. Either way, knowing the trade-offs — and asking your doctor which option makes sense for you — helps you save time, stress, and avoid procedures you may not need. Ultimately, a Radiologist's skill is critical. Specialists trained in mpMRI interpret scans about 25% more accurately.[38]

Misdiagnosis: What It Can Cost—and How to Protect Yourself

Even with today's advanced tests and imaging, mistakes still happen. And when they do, the consequences can be life-changing.

Take Paul's story. At 64, he was a careful businessman and father who took pride in weighing risks before making decisions. But when his PSA came back at 6.8 and his biopsy was flagged as *Gleason 7* — an "aggressive" cancer — he didn't ask for a second opinion. His urologist urged immediate surgery, warning about possible spread to his bones or lymph nodes.

Paul trusted the expert. He went through the surgery. Afterward, he faced incontinence that disrupted his work and personal life, leaving him ashamed and frustrated. Months later, a re-review of his biopsy revealed the truth: his cancer was actually *Gleason 6* — a low-risk form that likely did not require surgery at all. A simple second opinion might have saved him from regret.

Paul's case is far from rare. Research shows that when biopsy slides are re-examined by expert pathologists, approximately one in three diagnoses are changed — sometimes upgraded and sometimes downgraded. Another study found that nearly half of men initially labeled *"high risk"* were downgraded after surgery, proving that first impressions often make the cancer look worse than it is.[39] These errors are not harmless. They can push men into treatments they may not truly need — surgery, radiation, or hormone therapy — exposing them to lasting side effects such as incontinence or erectile dysfunction. Beyond the physical toll, these mistakes can rob men of peace of mind and quality of life.

When to Always Get a Second Opinion

- **After a biopsy report.** Pathological grades can differ; a re-read may change your diagnosis.

- **Before major treatment.** Decisions about surgery or radiation should never rest on a single voice.
- **When told it's "Urgent."** With Gleason 6, especially, surveillance is often a safe option. A second opinion can confirm whether waiting is the wiser course of action.

How to Put This into Action

If your biopsy shows cancer, request a second pathology review. Another pathologist may grade it differently, altering your entire treatment plan. Before undergoing surgery, radiation, or any major treatment, consider consulting a high-volume center or a prostate cancer specialty clinic for evaluation. Reviews like these frequently prevent overtreatment and spare men from procedures they never needed.

And don't worry about offending your doctor. Most urologists respect — even encourage — a second opinion. It shows you're taking your health seriously.

Real men have avoided regret by taking this step:

- A 70-year-old who was told surgery was "urgent" sought a second opinion; it confirmed surveillance was safe. "I kept my quality of life," he said with relief.
- A 62-year-old carpenter was told he had *Gleason 8* cancer. A second review corrected it to *Gleason 6*, sparing him unnecessary radiation.

The common thread? *The courage to ask for another set of eyes.*

The Bottom Line

Misdiagnosis can steal both health and peace of mind. A second opinion is your shield — the simplest, most powerful way to protect yourself from rushed or mistaken decisions. It can be the difference between a compromised life and a preserved one.

Actionable Items

- ✓ **Before a PSA Test:** Avoid cycling, sex, or heavy exercise for 48 hours.

- ✓ **After an Elevated PSA:** Repeat the test under the same conditions and track changes (PSA velocity).

- ✓ **At the Appointment:** Ask if the results could be from BPH or prostatitis instead of cancer.

5. **Imaging Choice:** Ask if mpMRI is available and covered; if not, request PSA density by ultrasound.

6. **If Cancer is Found:** Request a second pathology review and always get a second opinion, especially if told it's "Urgent."

- ✓ **For caregivers:** Support with prompts like, "*Should we reconfirm this diagnosis?*"

Preparing for a Biopsy — 10 Key Questions:

☐ Which approach will be used (transrectal or transperineal)?

☐ What's the infection risk?

☐ Will I have local or general anesthesia?

- ☐ How many samples will you take?
- ☐ What's the chance of missing cancer (false negatives)?
- ☐ Will I need antibiotics?
- ☐ How soon will results be ready?
- ☐ Who reviews the slides—are they specialists?
- ☐ What if results are inconclusive?
- ☐ Can MRI reduce the need for biopsy?

Key Takeaways

- **PSA is a clue, not a verdict.** Both high and "normal" results can mislead.

- **Four pitfalls drive confusion.** False positives, false negatives, everyday spikes, and no clue about tumor aggression.

- **Trends beat snapshots.** PSA velocity (rate of change) often matters more than a single reading.

- **Biopsies are manageable.** Preparation and smart questions reduce fear and risk.

- **Imaging is a trade-off.** Ultrasound is more accessible; mpMRI is more accurate but costly/limited.

- **Second opinions protect you.** Pathology re-reads catch errors and prevent overtreatment

PART 2
THE HEALING PATH

CHAPTER 4
MEDICAL BREAKTHROUGHS: SURGERY, RADIATION, AND EMERGING THERAPIES

"The art of medicine consists of amusing the patient while nature cures the disease."
— ***Voltaire***

You've made it through the maze — PSA tests, imaging scans, second opinions, and the rollercoaster of uncertainty. Now you stand at the crossroads that every man with prostate cancer eventually faces: **choosing a treatment path.**

It feels like staring at road signs that all point in different directions:

- Surgery.
- Radiation.
- Emerging therapies.
- Or even waiting and watching.

And the questions hit you all at once:

- Will surgery take away my vitality?
- Will radiation save me without leaving scars I'll live with forever?

- Can I even afford these newer therapies — or access them where I live?

Here's the hopeful news: today's treatments are not the blunt tools of the past. Medical breakthroughs have made them far more precise, less invasive, and often more effective. Survival rates tell part of the story: nearly *98% of men live at least five years* after diagnosis, and about *95% live 15 years or more*, according to the *National Cancer Institute's SEER Program.*[24]

But survival is only one measure. Treatments come with risks — side effects like incontinence or erectile dysfunction, which studies show affect more than *80% of men* at some point.[40] No wonder these are the questions that keep men awake at night.

This chapter is about clarity. We'll walk through surgery, radiation, and cutting-edge therapies like immunotherapy, showing you what each option offers, what it costs — not just in terms of money, but also in terms of quality of life — and how to weigh the trade-offs.

Whether you're the man making the decision or the loved one standing beside him, this chapter will equip you to sidestep pitfalls like overtreatment, regret, or unnecessary suffering.

Let's begin with the option most men encounter first — and the one often surrounded by the most myths and fears: *surgery*.

Robotic Surgery

For many men, the word *surgery* sparks fear of long scars, weeks in bed, and lingering side effects. But today, robotic-assisted radical prostatectomy has rewritten that story. Using advanced tools like the Da Vinci Surgical System, this approach has become a cornerstone of modern prostate cancer care. For men facing the diagnosis, robotic surgery represents not just hope for cancer control, but also a smoother recovery and the chance at preserving quality of life.

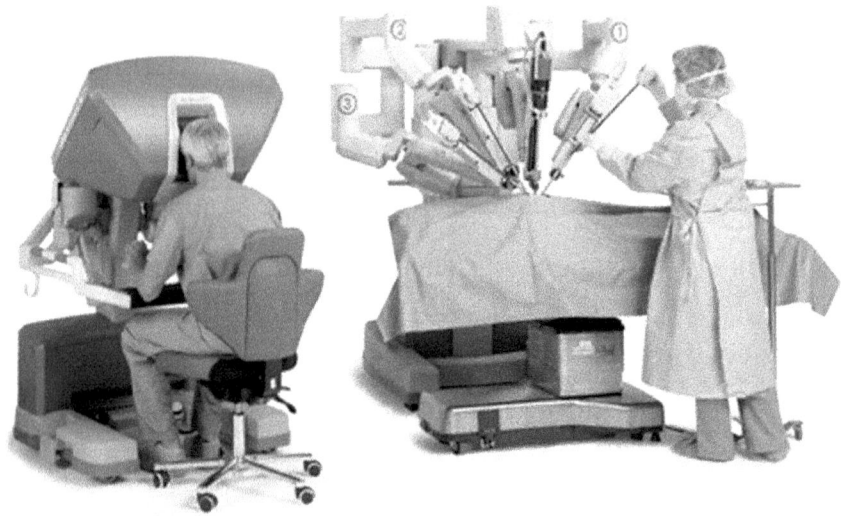

One of my patients, a 62-year-old retired mechanic, came to me dreading surgery. *"Doc, I can rebuild a carburetor blindfolded, but I can't rebuild my body if this goes wrong."* His fear was real — but so was his relief when he learned that robotic surgery often means smaller incisions, less pain, and a faster return to normal life. After his procedure, he walked out of the hospital in two days, joking that recovery was easier than fixing his old Chevy. His confidence stemmed from asking the right questions and knowing that there was a clear plan for both cancer treatment and recovery.

That's the promise of robotic surgery. Unlike traditional open surgery, which requires a large incision and a prolonged hospital stay, robotic-assisted procedures utilize small ports and highly precise instruments. Most men return home within one to two days, experiencing less pain and quicker healing.

A 2021 study in *JAMA Network Open* confirmed what patients like Martin experience: men who undergo robotic-assisted prostatectomy tend to recover faster, report less postoperative pain, and face fewer long-term issues like incontinence or erectile dysfunction.[41]

Still, the most common question every man asks is: *What will this mean for my sex life and bladder control?*

Understanding the Risks

Every man fears two things: intimacy and control. Erectile dysfunction (ED) remains the biggest worry. The good news is that nerve-sparing techniques, when possible, improve the odds of preserving function. However, the numbers remind us why preparation is crucial.

A 2016 review in the *World Journal of Men's Health* found[42]:

- Up to 68% of men report ED after surgery.
- Younger, healthier men with strong function before surgery recover more quickly.
- Nerve-sparing and robotic techniques improve the odds of success.
- Rehabilitation and medications (Viagra or similar drugs) often support recovery.

The truth is: outcomes vary. Factors such as pre-existing sexual health, tumor aggressiveness, and whether surgeons can safely preserve nerves all shape recovery.

Urinary incontinence is the second major concern. A *Johns Hopkins Report* found that about 10–15% of men still experience frequent leakage and need pads until six months after surgery, but fewer than 10% report using pads by three years.[43] Encouragingly, most men show steady improvement during the first year, especially with pelvic floor exercises and consistent follow-up care.

Nerve-Sparing

Cancers in the outer "peripheral zone" are often easier to treat while protecting nerves. Tumors closer to the center may force surgeons to sacrifice nerves for complete cancer control. This delicate balance — cancer removal versus quality of life — is why honest conversations with your surgeon matter. Knowing your tumor's location gives you the power to make informed choices.

What to Ask Before Surgery?

Technology helps, but a surgeon's experience is still the most significant predictor of success. Research in *BMC Urology* indicates that hospitals performing more than 100 robotic prostatectomies annually achieve better outcomes, including safer operations, shorter surgical times, and reduced blood loss.[44]

Before you decide, ask your surgeon these five questions:

1. How many robotic prostatectomies have you performed?
2. What is your nerve-sparing success rate?
3. What is your incontinence rate after surgery?
4. Do you use advanced imaging such as 3D mapping or MRI fusion to plan surgeries?
5. If my cancer is near the nerves, how will you balance cancer control with quality of life?

One of my patients, a 62-year-old retired mechanic, said these questions gave him peace of mind: *"It wasn't just about the surgeon's technical skill but knowing there was a thoughtful plan for my recovery."*

Robotic-assisted radical prostatectomy is a remarkable blend of technology and human expertise. With an experienced surgeon and the right questions, it can transform what was once a frightening ordeal into a carefully guided step toward healing and recovery.

Key Takeaway:

Surgery can always be daunting, but preparation through knowledge and open dialogue can turn fear into focus. The goal is not only to remove cancer, but also to protect dignity, function, and quality of life for years to come.

Radiation Therapy

When men hear "radiation," many picture old, harsh treatments that leave them weak and drained. But prostate cancer radiation therapy has changed dramatically in the last two decades. Today, it stands shoulder-to-shoulder with surgery as one of the most effective and widely used options. At its core, radiation works by aiming focused energy beams at the prostate to destroy cancer cells while sparing as much healthy tissue as possible. Thanks to modern breakthroughs, patients now have access to safer treatments, fewer side effects, and more flexible schedules than ever before.

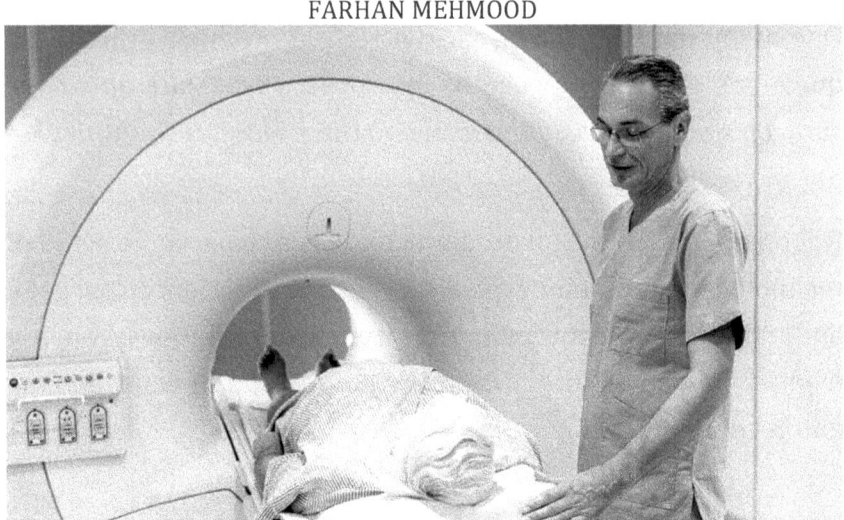

I remember speaking with Alan, a 60-year-old accountant, who dreaded the idea of sitting in a treatment chair every day for months. "I can barely sit through tax season," he joked. Yet when he learned about newer, shorter-course radiation options, his shoulders relaxed. For him, the fear wasn't radiation itself — it was losing control of his life.

Historically, the standard approach was *external beam radiation therapy (EBRT)*. Men often went five days a week for eight or nine weeks. While effective, the older beams couldn't conform closely to the prostate, and nearby organs got caught in the crossfire. A *Johns Hopkins* report found that about 20% of patients developed bowel issues such as diarrhea or rectal irritation.[45]

The Rise of IMRT and SBRT

CRITERIA	IMRT	SBRT
TREATMENT DURATION	5–9 WEEKS (DAILY SESSIONS)	SEVERAL WEEKS
SIDE EFFECTS	LOWER (MORE FRACTIONATED)	HIGHER
COST	LOWER	HIGHER
PRECISION	HIGH	HIGH

Intensity-modulated radiation therapy (IMRT) marked a turning point in prostate cancer care. With advanced imaging and computer guidance, IMRT can shape beams like a sculptor working in clay. This precision spares the bladder and rectum, and has kept bowel side effects to approximately 5% at two years, a significant improvement over older EBRT. [45]

Next came *Stereotactic Body Radiation Therapy (SBRT)*. SBRT compresses treatment into just five to seven sessions over one or two weeks. Despite the shorter course, outcomes are excellent. The 2024 PACE-B trial reported a five-year recurrence-free survival rate of about 95%, with fewer than 1% of men reporting bowel issues.[46] A 2018 *Journal of Clinical Oncology* study confirmed SBRT's side-effect profile was similar to IMRT, but often at a lower cost.[47]

So, what's the trade-off? IMRT typically means more visits but predictable insurance coverage. SBRT is faster and convenient but can be pricier, depending on where you live. For many men, the choice comes down to priorities: fewer trips to the clinic or lower long-term costs.

Proton Therapy

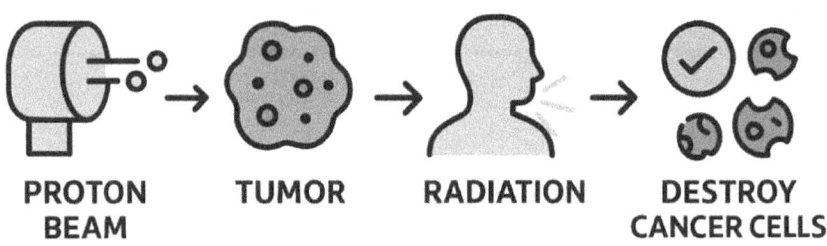

Proton therapy is the **new kid on the block.** Instead of X-rays, it uses charged particles that stop directly in the tumor, limiting collateral damage to nearby organs. For some men, this means fewer urinary or bowel side effects.

But there's a catch: *cost and access.* Treatments typically range from $50,000 to $100,000, and only about 40% of U.S. insurers cover it.[48] As of 2025, there are only 46 proton therapy centers in the United States. That makes it essentially an option for men living near major cities — or those willing to travel.[49]

Still, the results are promising. The Health Proton Therapy Institute did a study of more than 1,300 patients. They found that five years after treatment, three out of four high-risk men, and almost all low- and intermediate-risk men, were still cancer-free. Just as important, only a small number reported lasting side effects with their bladder or bowels.[50]

One patient, a 58-year-old teacher, told me he weighed proton therapy against IMRT. *"Proton looked fancy,"* he said, *"but IMRT worked, and it didn't break the bank."* His story highlights how cost, travel, and insurance coverage can influence decisions as much as clinical data.

Key Considerations When Choosing Your Radiation Therapy

Radiation therapy today often matches surgery in controlling localized prostate cancer. The right choice depends on your values and circumstances:

- **Access:** Is proton therapy available nearby, or are IMRT or SBRT more realistic?
- **Cost and Insurance:** What will insurance pay, and what's left for you?
- **Side Effects:** How much do urinary, bowel, or sexual risks shape your choice?
- **Lifestyle:** Do you prefer fewer, faster sessions (SBRT) or a longer, steady schedule (IMRT)?

A candid conversation with your oncologist is essential. Ask about success rates, potential side effects, and whether cutting-edge technologies like proton therapy offer real benefits for your specific cancer stage. Like Alan discovered, sometimes the right treatment is the one that not only fights cancer but also fits your life.

Key Insight:

Radiation therapy is no longer one-size-fits-all. IMRT, SBRT, and proton therapy offer strong cancer control with fewer side effects. The best choice depends on access, cost, side effects, lifestyle, and your goals with your medical team.

Immunotherapy and HIFU

Prostate cancer treatment has advanced rapidly over the past decade, and two of the most promising innovations are *immunotherapy* and *high-intensity focused ultrasound (HIFU)*. While not right for everyone, these treatments expand the toolbox, offering men who may not be ideal candidates for surgery or radiation new, more personalized paths. For many, they represent not just another therapy, but a chance to extend life or preserve quality of life where older treatments fall short.

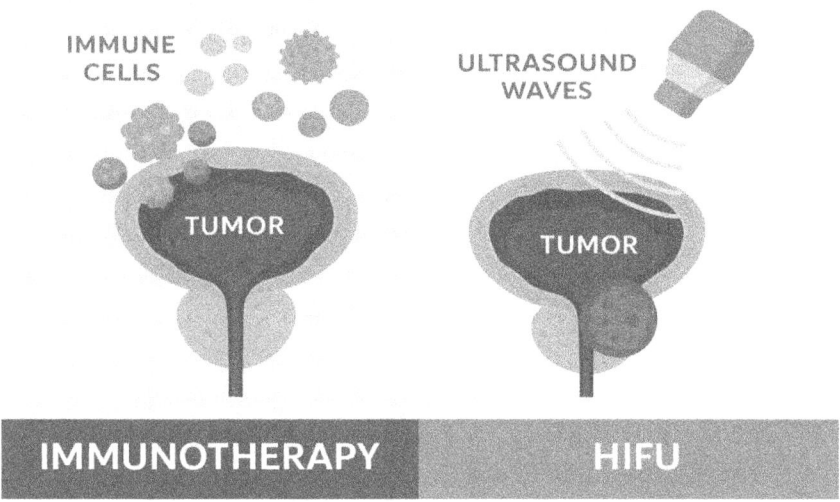

Immunotherapy

Unlike traditional treatments that directly attack tumors, immunotherapy trains the body's own immune system to do the work. One of the best-known options is *sipuleucel-T (Provenge)*, which involves collecting a man's immune cells, reprogramming them in the lab to better recognize prostate cancer, and then infusing them back.

One of the most studied therapies for prostate cancer is *sipuleucel-T (Provenge)*. This therapy involves taking a patient's immune cells, reprogramming them in a lab to identify prostate cancer more effectively, and then infusing them back into the body.

The results have been meaningful. In a pivotal *New England Journal of Medicine* trial (2010), men with advanced, castration-resistant prostate cancer lived a median of *25.8 months* with sipuleucel-T versus *21.7 months* with placebo — a 4.1-month gain that was statistically significant.[51]

But there's a catch: *cost.* A complete course involves three infusions over a month, totaling $90,000–$100,000, or about $30,000 per infusion.[51] Insurance coverage is inconsistent, leaving many men denied or burdened with high out-of-pocket bills.

For some, clinical trials offer hope. As of 2023, more than 500 prostate cancer immunotherapy trials were active across the United States, often providing access to cutting-edge treatments at reduced or no cost.[52]

One man I met — a 65-year-old retiree — joined such a trial after his insurer refused to cover him. *"It gave me hope when options were slim,"* he said. For him, the trial wasn't just about treatment; it was about reclaiming control and purpose.

HIFU

If immunotherapy is about boosting the body, *High-Intensity Focused Ultrasound (HIFU)* is about precision. Imagine a sniper's shot: sound waves heat and destroy only the cancer cells while sparing the rest of the prostate.

The appeal is obvious. Studies show that about 95% of men maintain urinary control and around 80% retain sexual function after HIFU— outcomes many find life-changing.[53]

Yet HIFU has limits. It is most effective for small, localized tumors and is often not covered by insurance. While research settings report costs around $1,100, in U.S. practice, men often face *$15,000–$25,000 per treatment.* Access is also limited, with only about 200 centers nationwide offering it.[54]

For the right patient, HIFU is powerful — but it isn't a universal cure. I recall a 59-year-old small business owner who considered HIFU. *"The numbers looked great,"* he said, *"but when I saw the cost and the travel, I had to step back."* He eventually pursued radiation closer to home — a reminder that practical factors, such as access and affordability, matter just as much as outcomes.

Key Questions to Ask Your Doctor

If you are considering either of these emerging therapies, it is crucial to have an open and informed conversation with your oncologist. Consider asking:

1. Am I eligible for these treatments based on my cancer stage and overall health?
2. Are there clinical trials that could give me access at lower or no cost?
3. What will insurance realistically cover, and what's my out-of-pocket responsibility?

The Bottom Line

Immunotherapy and HIFU are not universal solutions, but they are expanding what's possible in prostate cancer care. For some, they offer extended survival; for others, a way to preserve intimacy and control. Clinical trials often bridge the financial gap, ensuring that hope isn't limited to those who can pay out of pocket.

Modern medicine is moving steadily toward targeted, patient-centered care. By asking thoughtful questions and exploring every option, you can tailor your treatment plan not only to your diagnosis but also to your unique life circumstances.

When to Say No to Treatment?

Not every prostate cancer demands an immediate response. For some men, the wisest choice is to *wait and watch*. **Watchful waiting** — often recommended for older men with slow-growing disease — means monitoring symptoms without routine tests. **Active surveillance**, on the other hand, is a more structured approach for men with low-risk disease. It involves regular PSA tests, imaging, and occasional biopsies to ensure the cancer hasn't changed course.

The evidence is clear: many men with low-risk or carefully selected favorable intermediate-risk cancers (such as Gleason *3+4*) can be safely monitored without compromising long-term outcomes. In fact, adoption of active surveillance has climbed to about *60% among low-risk men in the U.S.*, reflecting this shift toward smarter, less invasive care.[55] Some men eventually move to treatment, either because of clinical changes or simply because anxiety made surveillance feel too stressful.

Five Red Flags of Overtreatment

- Gleason 6 with low PSA (<10) but rushed into surgery.
- No discussion of active surveillance.
- Treatment pushed without imaging.
- No second opinion offered.
- The doctor is treating other health risks instead of cancer itself.

Here's what this looks like in real life. A 60-year-old lawyer I spoke with was pressured into radiation for a Gleason 6 tumor. *"I felt bullied,"* he admitted. A second opinion changed everything. Instead of undergoing unnecessary radiation, he opted for active surveillance, thereby preserving both his health and quality of life. His story is a reminder: if your doctor skips alternatives, speak up and ask, *"Is active surveillance an option for me?"* Your care should be guided by your needs, not someone else's schedule.

The Bottom Line

Sometimes, saying *no* to treatment is not neglect — it's wisdom. For many men with low-risk prostate cancer, active surveillance protects quality of life without sacrificing safety.

And remember: choosing a treatment path doesn't have to feel like rolling dice. Robotic surgery offers precision but depends on a skilled surgeon. Modern radiation combines effectiveness with safety. New therapies, such as immunotherapy and HIFU, expand possibilities, although costs may limit access. And sometimes, waiting — patiently and carefully — is the most decisive move of all.

Think of the men we've met so far: the teacher who chose IMRT, the retiree who joined a clinical trial, and the lawyer who stood firm for surveillance. Each carved out a path that suited his circumstances. In the next chapter, we'll shift gears to nutrition — specifically, seven foods that research shows may help shrink tumors and complement any treatment plan.

You are not trapped at this crossroads. You are actively charting your own course.

Key Takeaways

- **Robotic surgery has transformed recovery.** Smaller incisions, less pain, faster healing—but surgeon skill is key.

- **ED and incontinence remain concerns.** Nerve-sparing techniques and pelvic floor rehab improve outcomes.

- **Radiation therapy evolved.** IMRT and SBRT offer precision with fewer side effects; proton therapy shows promise but is costly/less accessible.

- **Immunotherapy and HIFU expand options.** Particularly valuable for advanced cases or men unfit for surgery.

- **Avoid overtreatment.** Five red flags (including low-risk Gleason 6) mean treatment may do more harm than good.

- **Quality of life is as important as survival.** Choose treatment paths with dignity, function, and personal values in mind

CHAPTER 5

THE ANTI-CANCER DIET: 10 FOODS THAT SHRINK TUMORS

"Let food be thy medicine, and medicine be thy food."
— ***Hippocrates***

Imagine your body as a garden. Each cell is a plant: some thriving, others vulnerable to weeds. Food is the tool in your hand — with every bite, you can either nurture growth or feed disease. Prostate cancer, in particular, responds strongly to what you eat. The right foods, rich in protective compounds, can help slow tumor growth, strengthen the immune system, and reduce risk.

When 62-year-old Martin received his low-risk diagnosis, he felt powerless. Then his doctor suggested changing his diet. Within months, Martin had swapped fast food for salmon, spinach, and green tea. *"It made me feel like I was fighting back,"* he said. For Martin, food became more than fuel — it was empowerment.

In 2023, an estimated 288,300 U.S. men were diagnosed with prostate cancer. Research indicates that a plant-forward eating approach is associated with slower disease progression, whereas diets high in saturated fat are linked to worse outcomes.[56]

Whether you're managing a diagnosis, supporting a loved one, or focused on prevention, the right foods can help you reclaim control.

Foods to Fight Cancer

When it comes to fighting prostate cancer, your plate can be as powerful as a prescription. Decades of research have highlighted foods that help calm inflammation, support hormonal balance, and lower the risk of aggressive diseases. Here are ten everyday options backed by science. These foods don't promise a cure, but they arm your body with powerful defenses.

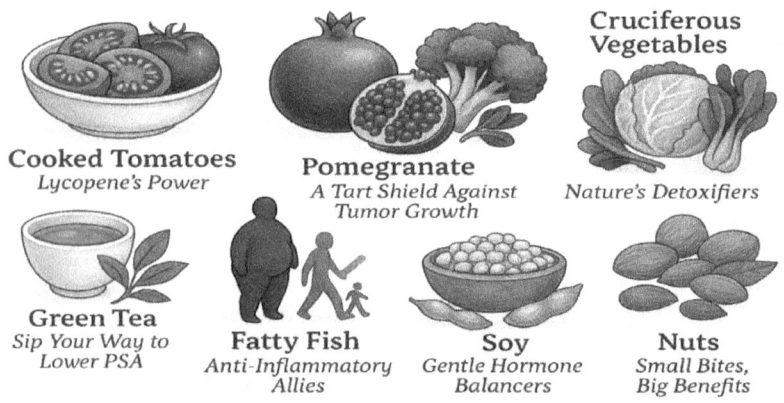

Cooked Tomatoes
Lycopene's Power

Pomegranate
A Tart Shield Against Tumor Growth

Cruciferous Vegetables
Nature's Detoxifiers

Green Tea
Sip Your Way to Lower PSA

Fatty Fish
Anti-Inflammatory Allies

Soy
Gentle Hormone Balancers

Nuts
Small Bites, Big Benefits

1. Cooked Tomatoes: Lycopene's Power

Tomatoes are packed with *lycopene*, a carotenoid that helps slow the growth of cancer cells. Here's the catch: *lycopene* is locked in the tomato's cell walls, and heat unlocks it. That's why cooked tomatoes — sauces, soups, and stews — pack more punch than raw ones.

- A cup of tomato sauce delivers ~20 mg of lycopene, a level linked with reduced aggressive prostate cancer risk.

- Men who consumed tomato products regularly were shown to have significantly lower rates of prostate cancer progression.[57]

Tip: Simmer marinara with olive oil (fat boosts absorption) and use it on whole-grain pasta, in soups, or as a base for curries.

2. Pomegranate: A Tart Shield Against Tumor Growth

Pomegranates are rich in ellagitannins — antioxidants known for their role in slowing prostate cancer progression. In one study, men who drank 8 oz of juice daily stretched their PSA doubling time from 15 months to 54 months.[58] In other words, their cancer was advancing three times more slowly.

Tip: Toss fresh seeds into salads, blend into smoothies, or drink unsweetened juice. Avoid sugary blends that dilute its power.

3. Cruciferous Vegetables: Nature's Detoxifiers

Broccoli, kale, Brussels sprouts, and other cruciferous vegetables carry sulforaphane and indole-3-carbinol — compounds that help neutralize toxins and coax unhealthy cells to shut down.[59]

Studies show that men who ate broccoli at least once a week had a 45% lower risk of developing aggressive prostate cancer.[60]

Tip: Steam lightly to preserve nutrients. Aim for half a cup daily — as a side dish, in stir-fries, or even blended into soups.

4. Green Tea: Sip Your Way to Lower PSA

Packed with catechins, green tea helps lower PSA levels and reduces the risk. In a Japanese study, men who drank five cups daily had a 48% lower risk of advanced cancer compared to those who drank less than one.[61]

Tip: Replace your afternoon coffee with green tea, brew iced batches for summer, or blend matcha powder into smoothies.

5. Fatty Fish: Omega-3 Allies

Salmon, sardines, and mackerel brim with *omega-3 fatty acids*, which fight inflammation — a known driver of cancer progression.

An *American Journal of Clinical Nutrition* meta-analysis found that men who ate fish regularly had a 63% lower risk of dying from prostate cancer compared to those who rarely ate fish.[62]

Tip: Bake, grill, or even use canned sardines. Aim for 2–3 servings weekly for both prostate and heart health.

6. Soy: Gentle Hormone Balancers

Soy foods, such as tofu, tempeh, and edamame, contain isoflavones, plant estrogens that help mitigate the influence of testosterone on cancer growth. A meta-analysis showed men with the highest soy intake had a 26% lower risk of prostate cancer; non-fermented soy (tofu, soymilk, edamame) had the most substantial effect.[63]

Tip: Add tofu to stir-fries, snack on roasted edamame, or switch to soy milk in your coffee.

7. Nuts: Small Bites, Big Benefits

Walnuts, almonds, pistachios, and pecans are packed with vitamin E, healthy fats, and antioxidants. In the *Health Professionals Follow-Up Study*, men with prostate cancer who ate nuts 5+ times per week had a 34% lower risk of dying from any cause compared with those who rarely consumed them.[64]

Tip: Snack on a handful daily, sprinkle over oatmeal, or blend into smoothies for staying power.

8. Berries: Polyphenol Powerhouses

Blueberries, raspberries, and strawberries are rich in anthocyanins, antioxidants that help reduce oxidative stress.

Studies show that berry polyphenols slow inflammatory pathways, helping the body become less hospitable to cancer growth.

Tip: Add a cup of mixed berries to your breakfast or blend them into smoothies for an antioxidant boost.

9. Whole Grains: Fiber as Defense

Oats, brown rice, and quinoa provide fiber that helps regulate insulin and lower hormone levels associated with cancer progression.

Tip: Swap white bread and pasta for whole-grain versions and add quinoa or farro to salads.

10. Turmeric: The Golden Protector

This golden spice contains *curcumin*, one of the most researched anti-cancer compounds. It blocks inflammatory pathways, slows tumor growth, and reduces oxidative stress.

Tip: Pair turmeric with black pepper (which boosts absorption 20-fold) and add it to curries, soups, or warm "golden milk."

The Takeaway

Food won't replace treatment, but it can shape your body's terrain — making it less hospitable to cancer. By weaving these ten foods into daily meals, you're not just eating — you're actively training your body to resist disease.

Martin's story reminds us that diet isn't just about survival; it's about regaining a sense of control. And when cancer tries to take that away, even a small, conscious choice — like swapping fries for a handful of walnuts — can feel like reclaiming power.

7-Day Prostate-Healing Meal Plan

Putting these cancer-fighting foods into action is easier than most people think. You don't need a chef's kitchen or exotic ingredients — just a few smart swaps and a willingness to experiment. This 7-day sample menu is built around ten of the most researched prostate-protective foods: tomatoes, broccoli, kale, salmon and other oily fish, tofu or soy, pomegranate, green tea, nuts, whole grains, and turmeric.

Think of this plan as a flexible blueprint rather than a rigid prescription. Each day combines at least three of these foods, giving your body a steady stream of protective compounds. And don't overlook your spice rack: *turmeric with black pepper* is a simple, affordable addition that research shows can slow tumor growth by targeting multiple cancer pathways.

Day-by-Day Breakdown

Here's what your weekly meal plan looks like:

Day 1

- *Breakfast:* Green tea with oatmeal topped with chopped walnuts.
- *Lunch:* Grilled salmon with lightly steamed broccoli.
- *Dinner:* Whole-wheat pasta tossed in tomato sauce and fresh spinach.
- *Snack:* Fresh pomegranate seeds.

Why it works: Omega-3s in salmon calm inflammation, lycopene in tomatoes slows cancer growth, and walnuts add antioxidant protection.

Day 2

- *Breakfast:* Soymilk smoothie blended with almonds.
- *Lunch:* Kale salad topped with crisp tofu cubes.
- *Dinner:* Baked mackerel with roasted Brussels sprouts dusted with turmeric.
- *Snack:* A soothing cup of green tea.

Why it works: Cruciferous veggies like Brussels sprouts detox harmful compounds, while soy gently balances hormones.

Day 3

- *Breakfast:* Green tea with yogurt and walnuts.
- *Lunch:* Hearty tomato soup with whole-grain bread.
- *Dinner:* Tofu stir-fry with broccoli, peppers, and carrots, seasoned with turmeric and black pepper.
- *Drink:* A glass of pomegranate juice.

Why it works: Lycopene-rich tomatoes, sulforaphane in broccoli, and curcumin in turmeric form a triple threat against tumor growth.

Day 4

- *Breakfast:* Soy yogurt with chopped almonds.
- *Lunch:* Salmon and kale salad with a squeeze of lemon.
- *Dinner:* Tomato-based vegetable curry with turmeric and pepper, served over brown rice.
- *Snack:* Green tea.

Why it works: Kale provides indole-3-carbinol for hormone balance, while curry spices add potent anti-inflammatory support.

Day 5

- *Breakfast:* Green tea with oatmeal topped with pomegranate seeds.
- *Lunch:* Warm broccoli and tofu soup.
- *Dinner:* Grilled mackerel with roasted cauliflower.
- *Snack:* A handful of walnuts.

Why it works: Pomegranate extends PSA doubling time, while crucifers like broccoli and cauliflower help neutralize carcinogens.

Day 6

- *Breakfast:* Soymilk smoothie with walnuts.
- *Lunch:* Tomato and kale salad with flakes of salmon.

- *Dinner:* Roasted Brussels sprouts with tofu, sprinkled with turmeric and black pepper.
- *Snack:* Green tea.

Why it works: This combination delivers antioxidants, omega-3s, and phytonutrients in one powerful day.

Day 7

- *Breakfast:* Green tea with yogurt and almonds.
- *Lunch:* Pomegranate-glazed chicken with steamed broccoli.
- *Dinner:* Whole-wheat tomato pasta with wilted spinach.
- *Snack:* Walnuts.

Why it works: Even lean proteins like chicken can pair with prostate-protective foods for balance and variety.

Budget-Friendly Shopping List

One of the best aspects of this plan is its affordability. With just a little planning, you can cover a week's worth of prostate-protective meals in under $50:

- Tomatoes (canned or fresh): $7 for 10 servings
- Frozen broccoli: $3 per pound
- Fresh kale: $2.50 per bunch
- Canned salmon: $5 per serving
- Tofu: $2 per block
- Green tea: $3 per box
- Walnuts: $5 per pound

- Pomegranate juice: $5 per liter
- Turmeric: $2 per jar
- Black pepper: $2 per jar

Food as Empowerment

I recall a 60-year-old caregiver who followed a similar plan with her husband. *"It was simple and gave us hope,"* she said. *"We felt like we were fighting back at the dinner table."* Their story is a reminder that healing meals aren't about perfection — they're about small, consistent choices that add up.

This plan is practical, affordable, and rooted in science. Even if you start small — sprinkling turmeric on roasted vegetables or trading white pasta for whole wheat — you're stacking the odds in your favor. Every plate becomes more than a meal. It becomes part of your healing.

Supplements that Work

Supplements can be part of your prostate health toolkit — but only if you choose wisely. The truth? The supplement aisle is crowded with flashy promises and miracle claims. Yet, only a few nutrients stand up to objective scientific evidence. The key is separating the hype from the helpful.

Let's focus on *three options* that have the best evidence and practical use, so you can make confident, informed decisions.

1. Saw Palmetto: The Classic Choice

Saw palmetto extract, made from the berries of the Serenoa repens plant, has long been used to ease urinary symptoms in men with an enlarged prostate (BPH).

- **What Research Says:** A 2020 *Cochrane* review found mixed results. Some studies have shown improved urinary flow and fewer nighttime bathroom trips, while others have found no significant difference compared to a placebo.[65] Quality matters here: standardized extracts (containing 85–95% fatty acids and sterols) consistently outperform cheaper formulations.

- **Other Perks:** Saw palmetto may also block the enzyme 5-alpha-reductase, which converts testosterone into DHT — a hormone linked to both prostate enlargement and hair loss.

- **A Real Story:** Mark, 67, tried a high-quality saw palmetto supplement after years of broken sleep. Within three months, he reported he was sleeping through the night again. *"It wasn't a miracle,"* he said, *"but it made life easier."*

Bottom line: Saw palmetto may not help with Prostate Cancer, but it can help reduce nighttime trips.

2. Beta-Sitosterol: The Quiet Contender

Imagine a plant-derived molecule that looks a lot like cholesterol — but acts like a light switch, dimming signals that cancer cells use to grow. That's beta-sitosterol in action.

In laboratory and animal studies, beta-sitosterol has been shown to induce apoptosis (programmed cell death) in prostate cancer cells, reduce invasiveness, and slow tumor progression. In benign prostate enlargement (BPH), it has helped improve urinary symptoms.[66]

Here's a useful way to see it: Think of testosterone as fuel, and dihydrotestosterone (DHT) as its turbocharged form. Beta-sitosterol can interfere with the enzyme that converts testosterone into DHT (5α-reductase), thereby reducing DHT's ability to stimulate prostate tissue growth.

What It Can (and Can't) Do for You

- It may improve urinary flow and reduce lower urinary tract symptoms (LUTS) in men with prostate enlargement, though not as powerfully as prescription drugs.

- It acts gently, with low risk of side effects — making it suitable for men wanting a milder approach before drugs.

- It has not been proven to treat prostate cancer or replace standard therapies. Its tumor-fighting effects, although promising in vitro and in animals, have not been reliably demonstrated in human clinical trials.

A Real-World Lens

One of my patients, a 59-year-old teacher, asked whether he should try beta-sitosterol before jumping to medication. We agreed — he trialed a high-quality, standardized form, monitored his urinary symptoms and PSA. Over the course of six months, his urinary frequency eased slightly, although his PSA level remained stable. He told me, *"It's not magic, but I prefer to start gentler before moving to harsh treatments."*

How to Use It Wisely

- Look for **standardized extracts**, not vague "proprietary blends."

- Combine with evidence-backed lifestyle steps (diet, movement, sleep).

- Monitor your results (urinary scores, PSA, side effects) over 3–6 months.

- Always check with your doctor — it can interact with other medications.

Bottom Line: Beta-sitosterol is not a cure, but it's a scientifically grounded option worth considering when symptoms are mild and a gentler approach is desired. Used smartly and cautiously, it may alleviate urinary discomfort without resorting to pharmaceuticals.

3. The Blend Approach

ProstaVive is one of the newer multi-ingredient supplements. It combines vitamins and minerals (zinc, magnesium, and vitamin D) with herbs such as tongkat ali, ashwagandha, fenugreek, ginseng, maca root, and nettle root.

What research says: While the full formula hasn't been clinically tested, many of its individual ingredients have evidence for supporting prostate or sexual health. For example, zinc is essential for sperm production and hormone balance, vitamin D supports immune health, and nettle root has been shown in some studies to reduce urinary symptoms.

The catch: Proprietary blends often don't list exact dosages, making it hard to know how much of each nutrient you're getting.

A real story: One retiree told me ProstaVive left him with more energy and fewer nighttime bathroom trips, but admitted, *"It's hard to know which part of it helped — and it wasn't cheap."*

Bottom line: ProstaVive may be beneficial if the budget allows, but consider it an add-on, not a substitute for proven approaches.

The Doctor's Take

Supplements can play a role, but they're not magic bullets. Think of them as **supporting actors**, not the star of the show.

- **Start with lifestyle first:** A diet rich in tomatoes, cruciferous veggies, green tea, fish, soy, nuts, and turmeric will always do more for your prostate than any capsule.

- **Choose wisely:** If you want to try supplements, saw palmetto and beta-sitosterol have the most credible track records. Blends like ProstaVive can help save you the hassle of mixing multiple ingredients.

- **Talk with your doctor:** Supplements can interact with medications, especially blood thinners. Never start a new regimen without consulting your doctor first.

- **The key message?** Don't buy the hype. Use supplements as *tools, not as a cure*. When paired with a prostate-healing diet, regular exercise, and evidence-based medical care, the right supplement can support your journey.

Case Example: John's Turnaround

John, a 57-year-old truck driver, had spent decades on the road fueled by fast food and cola. When his doctor diagnosed him with *high-grade prostatic intraepithelial neoplasia (PIN)* — a precancerous condition tied to increased prostate cancer risk — his elevated PSA levels made the warning all too real. John admitted later, "I thought my lifestyle had finally caught up with me."

Determined to change course, John embraced a prostate-protective routine. His mornings started with oatmeal topped with walnuts, swapping out sugary pastries. Lunch consisted of broccoli and tofu salads, and dinner featured salmon simmered in tomato sauce with turmeric and black pepper — a nutrient-rich plate filled with lycopene, omega-3 fatty acids, and curcumin. Blood tests also revealed vitamin D deficiency, so under his doctor's guidance, he began supplementing with *2,000 IU daily*. To round out the changes, John replaced soda with green tea twice a day and made time for 30-minute walks after long periods of inactivity.

A year later, the payoff was undeniable. His PSA stabilized, his energy improved, and a follow-up biopsy revealed no progression of PIN. John's experience mirrored findings from clinical research: in a one-year trial of men with high-grade PIN, only *3%* of those taking daily green tea catechins developed prostate cancer, compared with *30%* in the placebo group. Just as important, no significant side effects were noted.

John's story is more than anecdote — it is living proof of what research is beginning to confirm. Food, lifestyle, and targeted supplements are not magic bullets, but they shift the odds in your favor. Combined with regular medical care, they offer men not just protection but empowerment. For John, the shift from burgers and soda to a nutrient-rich, evidence-based plan didn't just change his lab results — it changed his outlook. He moved from fear of disease to confidence in his future.

Key Takeaways

- **Food is your first medicine.** A plant-forward diet rich in tomatoes, crucifers, soy, and walnuts helps lower inflammation, balance hormones, and protect the prostate.
- **Small swaps make a big impact.** Replacing soda with green tea or chips with walnuts shifts your body's chemistry toward healing.
- **Supplements can help—but wisely.** Evidence supports targeted options, such as **beta-sitosterol** (urinary health), **zinc** (hormones & prostate tissue), and **vitamin D** (immune & bone strength). Others are overhyped and lack proof.
- **Whole foods > pills.** No supplement can replace the synergy of a balanced, anti-inflammatory diet.
- **Doctor first, bottle second.** Always review supplements with your oncologist to avoid drug interactions and wasted money.
- **Consistency beats complexity.** Building simple daily food routines (broccoli at lunch, tomatoes 3x a week, green tea daily) is far more effective than chasing miracle products.

Lifestyle + nutrition = synergy. When paired with stress management and physical activity, smart eating and evidence-based supplements can amplify healing and resilience.

FARHAN MEHMOOD
BONUS GIFT
TOP 7 FOODS FOR A HEALTHY PROSTATE

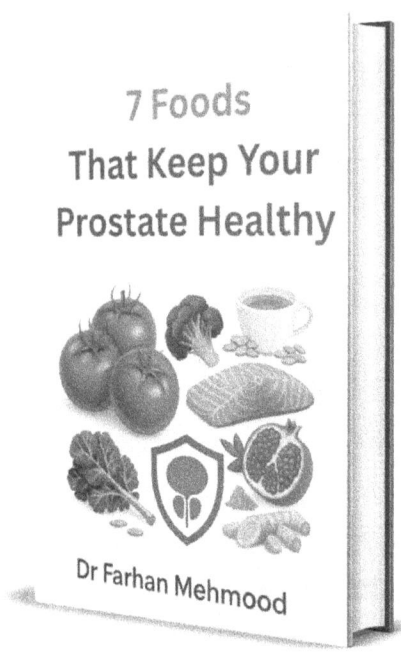

You've just finished Chapter 5 and already learned how powerful nutrition can be for your prostate. Now it's time to take the next step and get your FREE printable guide **(Scan the QR Code Above).**

This quick reference will show you:
- ✓ The antioxidant-rich foods proven to reduce prostate inflammation.
- ✓ The superfood that helps balance hormones and support urinary flow.
- ✓ The best drink for long-term prostate protection.
- ✓ 3 easy swaps to improve your daily diet — instantly.

CHAPTER 6
ALTERNATIVE THERAPIES THAT WORK (AND THE SCAMS TO AVOID)

"Beware of false knowledge; it is more dangerous than ignorance."
— *George Bernard Shaw*

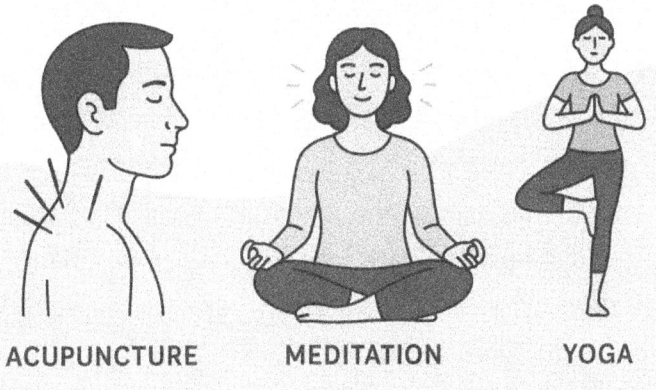

Imagine strolling through a crowded marketplace. Vendors are shouting at you from every corner. One waves a bottle of pills claiming to *"cure cancer naturally."* Another insists their herbal tea will *"lower PSA in 30 days."* In the distance, a quieter stall offers yoga mats, acupuncture needles, and a pamphlet titled *Integrative Oncology.*

If you're a man living with prostate cancer, this scene may feel all too familiar. Ads pop up on your phone. Friends forward miracle cures they've read about online. And in late-night moments of fear, Google serves up promises of secret remedies that sound almost believable.

I once worked with two men who illustrate the split that happens in this marketplace of hope.

The first, a 64-year-old accountant, invested in an overseas program offering *"miracle teas"* and detox regimens. He spent thousands of dollars and six months of precious time drinking herbal concoctions. His PSA kept rising, and his biopsy showed his cancer had progressed. *"I thought I was buying time,"* he later told me, *"but I was only buying false hope."*

The second man, 61 and newly retired, took a different route. He signed up for acupuncture sessions at his cancer center, joined a beginner's yoga class, and began a daily mindfulness routine. Within weeks, he noticed he was sleeping better, his hot flashes from hormone therapy were easing, and his anxiety had softened. *"I didn't cure my cancer with yoga,"* he laughed, *"but I cured the fear that came with it."*

This is the crossroads many men face: do you spend time and money chasing miracle cures, or do you invest in evidence-based therapies that may not eradicate cancer but can absolutely improve the way you live with it?

This chapter is about separating science from salesmanship. It's about arming yourself with the knowledge to choose therapies that truly support your recovery and spotting the red flags that signal scams.

Why Men Seek Alternatives?

A prostate cancer diagnosis changes everything. Suddenly, your calendar fills with PSA tests, biopsies, MRIs, and appointments with surgeons or radiation oncologists. The words "erectile dysfunction" and "incontinence" creep into conversations you never thought you'd have.

For many men, the fear isn't just about cancer itself — it's about losing control over their body, their masculinity, and their independence. That's when the lure of alternative therapies kicks in.

- **Fear of Side Effects**: Surgery and radiation save lives, but they carry real risks. Who wouldn't be tempted by a natural therapy that claims to heal without harm?

- **Desire for Control**: Cancer often makes men feel like passengers in their own lives. Choosing an alternative therapy can restore a sense of agency.

- **The "Natural" Appeal**: We're wired to believe that if something comes from nature, it must be safe. But as you'll see, "natural" doesn't always mean harmless.

Seeking more than what standard medicine offers isn't foolish — it's human. The challenge is knowing where to draw the line between supportive therapies and dangerous distractions.

Complementary vs. Alternative: The Critical Distinction

One of the biggest mistakes men make is confusing complementary therapies with alternative therapies. The words sound similar, but the consequences are not.

- **Complementary therapies** are used alongside medical care. They aim to ease symptoms, reduce stress, and improve quality of life. Examples: acupuncture for pain, yoga for fatigue, meditation for anxiety, or hyperthermia to boost the effect of radiation.

- **Alternative therapies** are used instead of medical treatment. This is where danger lies. Relying solely on an unproven herbal remedy or miracle supplement while delaying surgery, radiation, or hormone therapy can allow cancer to progress unchecked.

The golden rule is simple: *Complement, don't replace.*

If a therapy fits naturally alongside your medical care, has been studied in credible trials, and is offered at reputable cancer centers, it's worth exploring. If it promises to cure cancer without surgery, radiation, or medication, walk away.

How to Judge What's Credible

Here's where many men get tripped up. An article online sounds convincing. A friend swears by a supplement. A video promises, "Big Pharma doesn't want you to know." How do you know what's worth your time — and what's a scam?

Here are four filters you can use:

1. **Check the Source.** Is the therapy backed by peer-reviewed clinical trials, or is it supported only by testimonials? Anecdotes make good stories, but they are poor evidence.

2. **Follow the Experts.** Do reputable cancer centers — Johns Hopkins, Mayo Clinic, MD Anderson — offer it as part of integrative care? If yes, that's a strong signal.

3. **Ask Your Doctor.** Could this therapy interact with your medications? A good oncologist won't dismiss everything "natural" but will help you evaluate safety.

4. **Look for Red Flags.** Phrases like *"100% cure rate,"* *"secret formula,"* or *"no side effects"* are clear warning signs. So are offshore-only clinics that demand thousands of dollars upfront.

Remember:
Hope is powerful, but hope without evidence can be dangerous and costly. Skip "miracle" supplements and unproven clinics. Save your resources for therapies and lifestyle changes that are rigorously tested and proven to help.

Mind-Body Healing — The Hidden Power

When men hear the word *cancer*, their mind often races faster than the disease itself. *"What if it spreads? What if I can't work? What if the treatment changes me?"* Stress becomes a silent second illness, fueling inflammation, disrupting hormones, and weakening the very immune system your body needs to fight back.

That's why mind-body therapies matter. They don't shrink tumors directly, but they can change the terrain in which cancer grows. Lower stress hormones, such as cortisol, help calm inflammation and steadier moods, giving your body a better chance to fight. Think of it this way: while surgery and radiation work on the battlefield, meditation and breathwork rebuild the fortress walls and supply lines.

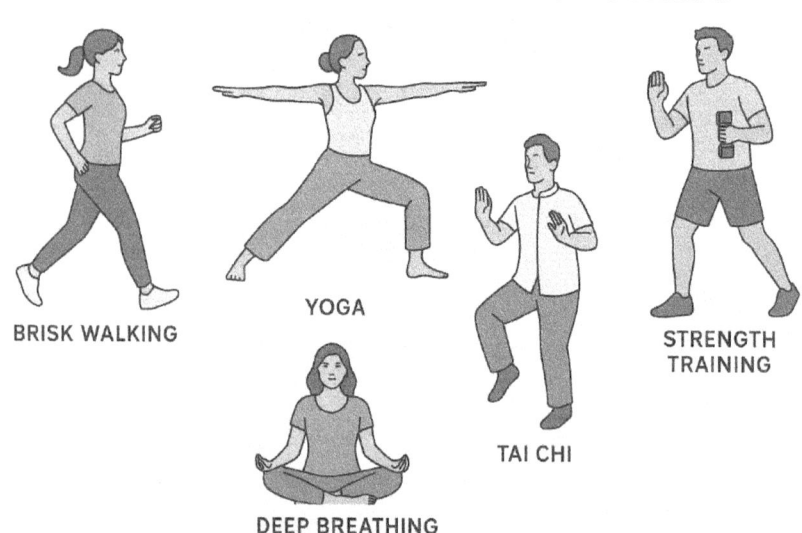

Meditation & Mindset: Training the Brain for Healing

A few years ago, I spoke with a 59-year-old engineer named Paul. After his diagnosis, he couldn't sleep. Every night, he'd stare at the ceiling, gripped by *"what if"* thoughts. His oncologist suggested guided meditation. Skeptical at first, Paul began with just 10 minutes a day, following an app on his phone. Within weeks, he noticed he was sleeping better, his blood pressure dipped, and he felt calmer during appointments. *"It didn't erase the cancer,"* he said, *"but it erased the fear that was eating me alive."*

That's the power of mindset.

Dr. Joe Dispenza, a researcher and author, has popularized the idea that meditation can actually *rewire* the brain. His approach combines neuroscience and mindfulness, teaching individuals to break free from survival-driven thought patterns and cultivate new habits of calmness, focus, and resilience. While some of his claims are debated, the core insight is supported by science: regular meditation reduces stress hormones, eases anxiety, and improves quality of life in cancer patients.

A 2022 randomized controlled trial in *Contemporary Clinical Trials* found that mindfulness-based stress reduction significantly lowered anxiety, depression, and fear of recurrence in prostate cancer survivors.[67]

Key Takeaways:

- Start with 10–15 minutes of guided meditation daily. Apps like Headspace, Calm, or free YouTube recordings can help.
- Focus on simple breath awareness or body scan techniques.
  If your mind wanders (and it will), gently bring it back — training the brain is like training a muscle.

- Meditation isn't about silencing thoughts; it's about changing your relationship with them. Over time, it can turn fear into focus and stress into strength.

Breathwork: Reclaiming Control, One Breath at a Time

If meditation feels too abstract, here's the good news: you can start with something as simple as breathing. Breath is the bridge between body and mind, and learning to control it can calm stress, reduce inflammation, and even sharpen immune function.

The most famous pioneer here is Wim Hof, known as *"The Iceman."* His method combines three pillars:

1. **Controlled breathing** (deep, rhythmic rounds).
2. **Cold exposure** (like cold showers or ice baths).
3. **Focused mindset.**

While plunging into an ice bath may not appeal to everyone, science is intriguing. Studies have shown that Hof-style breathwork reduces stress hormones, lowers inflammation, and increases resilience. A landmark 2014 study in *PNAS* found that participants practicing Hof's breathing techniques could voluntarily influence their immune response, reducing inflammatory markers after exposure to bacterial toxins.[68]

You don't need an ice river to benefit from it. Even simple breathwork practices can help men with prostate cancer manage stress and PSA anxiety:

- **Box breathing:** Inhale for 4 seconds, hold for 4, exhale for 4, hold for 4. Repeat for 5–10 minutes.

- **Hof-style rounds (gentle beginner version):** Take 30 deep breaths (in through the nose, out through the mouth), exhale fully, then hold until you feel the urge to breathe. Inhale deeply, hold for 10–15 seconds. Repeat 2–3 times.

One 63-year-old patient told me he used box breathing before every PSA test. "It stopped the panic spiral," he explained. "Instead of dreading the results, I walked in steady."

Key Takeaways:

- Start with 5–10 minutes of daily breathwork.
- Use box breathing before stressful appointments.
- Try one round of Hof-style breathing in the morning to energize your day.

Why This Matters?

Mind-body practices like meditation and breathwork may sound *"soft"* compared to the hard science of surgery or radiation, but research tells a different story. They lower cortisol, improve immune balance, reduce fatigue, and even boost quality of life scores in men with prostate cancer.

Real power lies in control. Cancer often makes men feel powerless. Meditation and breathwork hand back the steering wheel. With each session, you're not just calming your mind — you're shaping the internal environment in which healing happens.

Movement for Healing

When most men think of "exercise," they picture treadmills, weights, or long jogs. But when you're facing prostate cancer, the kind of movement that heals looks very different. Instead of pounding the pavement, it's about gentle, intentional motion — moving in ways that restore energy, reduce stress, and rebuild confidence in your body.

These practices aren't about six-pack abs. They're about strength where it matters: in your immune system, your pelvic floor, and your emotional resilience. Let's look at three powerful approaches: *yoga, tai chi, and qigong.*

Yoga: Strength and Stillness Combined

I once met a 64-year-old man, Daniel, who had just finished a round of radiation therapy. His biggest complaint wasn't pain — it was exhaustion. "I felt like my body's battery was stuck at 30%," he said. On his doctor's recommendation, he joined a yoga class at his cancer center. Within six weeks, he noticed less fatigue, better sleep, and even more confidence in the bedroom.

That story isn't unique. Research backs it up. A University of Pennsylvania trial found that men practicing yoga twice a week during radiation reported less fatigue, improved sexual function, and stronger emotional well-being compared to men who didn't. In fact, some participants even noted better bladder control, thanks to yoga's pelvic floor–strengthening effects.

Why Yoga Works?
- **Reduces fatigue** by improving blood flow and oxygenation.

- **Boosts sleep** by calming the nervous system.
- **Strengthens the pelvic floor** — key for regaining bladder control after surgery or radiation.
- **Supports erectile function** through improved circulation and reduced stress.

Practical Takeaways (how to start)

Aim for **2–3 sessions per week** (20–40 minutes). Begin with gentle, restorative poses:

- **Bridge pose** (strengthens the pelvic floor).
- **Cat-cow stretch** (loosens the spine and reduces tension).
- **Seated forward bend** (calms the nervous system and stretches the hamstrings).

Tip: Consider using a video, an app, or classes at a local cancer center — many now offer yoga specifically designed for survivors.

Tai Chi & Qigong: The Art of Gentle Energy

If yoga feels too stretchy or intimidating, tai chi and qigong offer another path. These ancient Chinese practices focus on slow, flowing movements paired with breath control. Think of it as "moving meditation."

A 2021 study in *Supportive Care in Cancer* found that cancer survivors who practiced tai chi experienced reduced stress, better sleep, and improved immune markers compared with those who didn't. Other trials have shown that qigong — a close cousin of tai chi — lowers fatigue and enhances overall quality of life during treatment.

Why Tai Chi & Qigong Work?

- Reduce stress by calming the autonomic nervous system.
- Improve circulation and balance — especially important if treatments leave you feeling weak or dizzy.
- Regulate hormones and immune function, supporting recovery.
- Offer a safe, low-impact option for men who can't manage traditional exercise.

Practical Takeaways (how to start)

Just *15 minutes a day* is enough. Free resources are abundant — YouTube videos, local community classes, or even guided DVDs designed for beginners and seniors.

Focus on simple routines like:

- **Tai chi "commencement form"** — a gentle opening stance with controlled breaths.
- **Qigong "lifting the sky"** — slowly raising your arms overhead while inhaling, lowering them as you exhale.

Integrative Medical Alternatives

When we think of "medicine," most of us picture pills, scans, or surgery. But modern cancer care is evolving. Today, the smartest approach isn't just choosing between Western and Eastern medicine — it's blending the best of both. These *integrative therapies* don't replace standard treatment, but they can ease side effects, improve recovery, and strengthen emotional resilience along the way.

Let's dive into three categories that are changing lives: *acupuncture, hyperthermia, and mind-body clinical support.*

Acupuncture: Small Needles, Big Relief

I once met Robert, a 61-year-old man struggling with hot flashes after hormone therapy. His nights were sleepless, and his energy tanked. A friend suggested acupuncture, and he was skeptical — "How could needles fix this?" But after six weeks of weekly sessions, he reported better sleep, fewer hot flashes, and an energy lift he hadn't felt in months.

Science backs him up. A 2024 trial in *Supportive Care in Cancer* showed that acupuncture improved sleep, fatigue, and quality of life in men with prostate cancer undergoing treatment.[69] Other studies confirm its benefits for urinary symptoms, pain, and hormone therapy–related hot flashes.

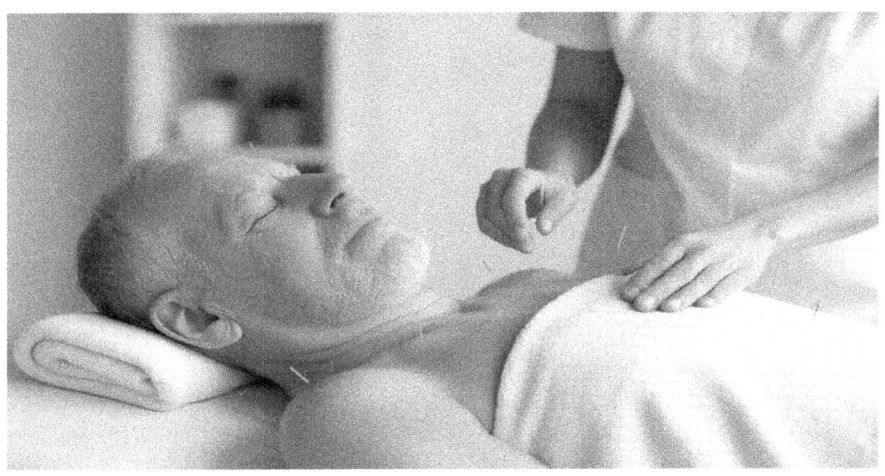

Practical Guide

- **Frequency:** Most men benefit from 1–2 sessions per week during treatment, then taper to monthly maintenance.
- **Cost:** $50–$100 per session. Some insurance plans (including Medicare in some instances) cover it.
- **Safety:** Always choose a licensed acupuncturist, ideally one affiliated with a cancer center.

Remember: If you're struggling with pain, fatigue, or hormone-related symptoms, acupuncture is one of the most evidence-backed complementary tools you can add to your care plan.

Hyperthermia: Turning Up the Heat on Cancer

Hyperthermia may sound futuristic, but the idea is simple: heat weakens cancer cells. By raising prostate tissue temperature to about 104–113°F (40–45°C), tumors become more vulnerable — especially to treatments like radiation.

In fact, a recent clinical trial found that adding hyperthermia to IMRT (intensity-modulated radiation therapy) improved treatment outcomes by about *20%* compared with radiation alone.[70] Patients not only had better tumor control but also tolerated the therapy well.

Availability & Access

- Roughly *50 centers in the U.S.* offer hyperthermia, mostly at major cancer hospitals.
- It's typically used as an adjunct, not a standalone therapy.

- Side effects are usually mild: temporary redness, warmth, or mild discomfort in the treated area.

Practical Takeaway

Ask your radiation oncologist if a nearby cancer center offers hyperthermia. For men with localized or high-risk tumors, it may buy time, enhance treatment effectiveness, and help delay the need for more aggressive interventions.

Mind-Body Clinical Support: Healing Beyond the Tumor

Cancer doesn't just attack the body; it shakes identity, emotions, and relationships. That's where mind-body therapies step in. Far from being "soft science," these tools have a measurable impact.

- **Music Therapy:** Studies show it reduces anxiety, lowers blood pressure, and improves mood during treatment. Something as simple as guided music sessions during chemotherapy can make the experience far less overwhelming.

- **Art Therapy:** For men who find it hard to talk about fear or frustration, drawing or painting provides an outlet that words can't.

- **Massage Therapy:** Beyond relaxation, massage has been shown to reduce pain, ease muscle tension, and improve sleep. In cancer centers, it's often integrated into supportive care for this reason.

A patient I worked with — a 58-year-old teacher — described massage therapy during his recovery as *"the one hour each week where I felt human again."* That sense of emotional release is as vital to healing as any medication.

Practical Steps

- Look for cancer centers that offer integrative programs (many now include acupuncture, massage, and music therapy).

- At home, consider guided music apps, community art classes, or relaxation massage with therapists trained in oncology care.

- Even one 30-minute session per week can improve stress, mood, and overall recovery.

Building Your Personal Healing Toolkit

When it comes to prostate cancer, the most powerful approach isn't choosing either medical care or alternative therapies — it's combining the two into a toolkit that supports your whole body. Think of it like building a home: doctors provide the foundation with treatments such as surgery or radiation, but you furnish the inside with practices that make daily life stronger, calmer, and more livable.

The key is harmony, not replacement. These practices are not meant to *replace* medical treatment. Instead, they help reduce side effects, lower stress, and give you a greater sense of control while you move through your care plan.

Here's how you can put it all together into a simple weekly routine.

A Sample Healing Week

Morning Reset

- **Breathwork:** Start with 10 minutes of controlled breathing. If you're new, try *box breathing* (inhale 4, hold 4, exhale 4, hold 4). More adventurous? Try one round of the *Wim Hof method* — 30 deep inhales, exhale, then hold until you feel the urge to breathe. This not only calms anxiety but also boosts oxygen flow and strengthens resilience.

- **Green Tea:** Swap your morning coffee for a cup of antioxidant-rich green tea. Catechins in green tea have been linked to lower PSA and slower cancer progression.

Afternoon Recharge

- **Yoga or Tai Chi (20–30 minutes):** Gentle poses like the bridge pose or cat-cow can strengthen the pelvic floor, reduce fatigue, and improve sexual function. If yoga feels intimidating, Tai Chi or Qigong are perfect alternatives — they're slow, flowing, and beginner-friendly. Evidence shows that even 15 minutes daily can lower stress and improve immune resilience.

- **Snack idea:** A handful of walnuts or pomegranate seeds — both linked to improved prostate health and longevity.

Evening Wind-Down

- **Meditation (10–15 minutes):** Stress fuels inflammation and hormonal imbalance. Guided meditations — like those by **Dr. Joe Dispenza** — teach you to rewire thought patterns, quiet anxiety, and build emotional resilience. Studies have shown that regular meditation lowers cortisol levels, improves sleep, and enhances the quality of life in cancer patients.

- **Gratitude journaling (optional):** Note one thing you're grateful for. Even this small act improves mood and reduces anxiety.

Weekly Reset

- **Acupuncture or Massage:** Schedule one session each week to address fatigue, pain, or hot flashes. If access is limited, massage therapy or guided relaxation at home can be beneficial.

- **Supplements:** Review any supplements with your oncologist. Stick to evidence-backed ones like vitamin D, zinc, or beta-sitosterol instead of chasing miracle pills.

Putting Everything into Practice

The toolkit doesn't demand perfection. You don't need to meditate every night or never miss a yoga class. The goal is *consistency, not rigidity*. Even stacking two or three of these habits most days can create a compounding effect over weeks and months.

Take Sam, a 64-year-old electrician I spoke with. After his diagnosis, he felt powerless. His doctor suggested standard radiation, but Sam wanted more control. He established a routine: practicing breathwork in the morning, attending yoga twice a week, switching to green tea instead of soda, and receiving weekly acupuncture. Six months later, his energy level was higher, his sleep was more profound, and his PSA levels had stabilized. *"I can't say it cured me,"* he told me, *"but it gave me back my life."*

That's the point of this toolkit. It's not about rejecting medicine or chasing unproven fads. It's about weaving safe, supportive therapies that make you feel stronger, calmer, and more in control — every single day.

Key Takeaways

- **Not all "natural cures" are equal.** Some therapies — like acupuncture, yoga, meditation, and hyperthermia — have credible research backing them. Others, like baking soda "cures" or apricot kernels, are harmful and should be avoided.

- **Complement, don't replace.** Safe alternative practices work best when paired with medical treatments, not as stand-alone "miracle" substitutes. Harmony, not exclusion, is the key.

- **Mind-body practices matter.** Meditation, breathwork, and mindset training lower stress hormones, improve resilience, and can enhance quality of life during treatment.

- **Movement heals.** Gentle exercises such as yoga, Tai Chi, or Qigong can reduce fatigue, strengthen the pelvic floor, improve sleep, and help restore sexual function.

- **Integrative therapies offer relief.** Acupuncture, massage, and music/art therapy can ease pain, hot flashes, and emotional stress. Hyperthermia shows promise as an adjunctive treatment.

- **Build your toolkit.** A weekly routine of breathwork, movement, meditation, supportive nutrition, and select therapies creates momentum and restores control..

PART 3
PREVENTION & LIFELONG HEALTH

CHAPTER 7
THE 90-DAY PROSTATE RESET

"A journey of a thousand miles begins with a single step."
— Lao Tzu

When Peter, a 61-year-old retired pilot, was first told his PSA had crept up, he did what many of us do: he tried everything at once. He bought supplements, downloaded five different diets, signed up for a yoga class, and promised to meditate daily. Within three weeks, he was exhausted, frustrated, and ready to give up.

What turned things around wasn't another *"miracle solution."* It was the structure. His oncologist suggested he focus on just one or two habits each week for 90 days. That's when change sticks. By the end of three months, Peter's PSA had stabilized, he was sleeping through the night, and, for the first time, he felt in control of his health again.

The truth is: you don't need perfection. You just need a plan. And that's precisely what this chapter offers: a *13-week roadmap* to rebuild prostate health—simple, structured, and backed by science.

However, this plan is **not meant to replace your doctor's advice**. Think of it as a companion to your medical care, not a substitute for it. You shouldn't follow it in isolation or abandon your healthcare provider's guidance—both go hand in hand for the best outcomes.

Why a Reset Works

Think of your body like a system that's been overloaded. Years of stress, poor diet, irregular sleep, and neglect add up, and prostate health often takes the hit. A reset is about hitting pause, recalibrating, and giving your body and mind a chance to heal.

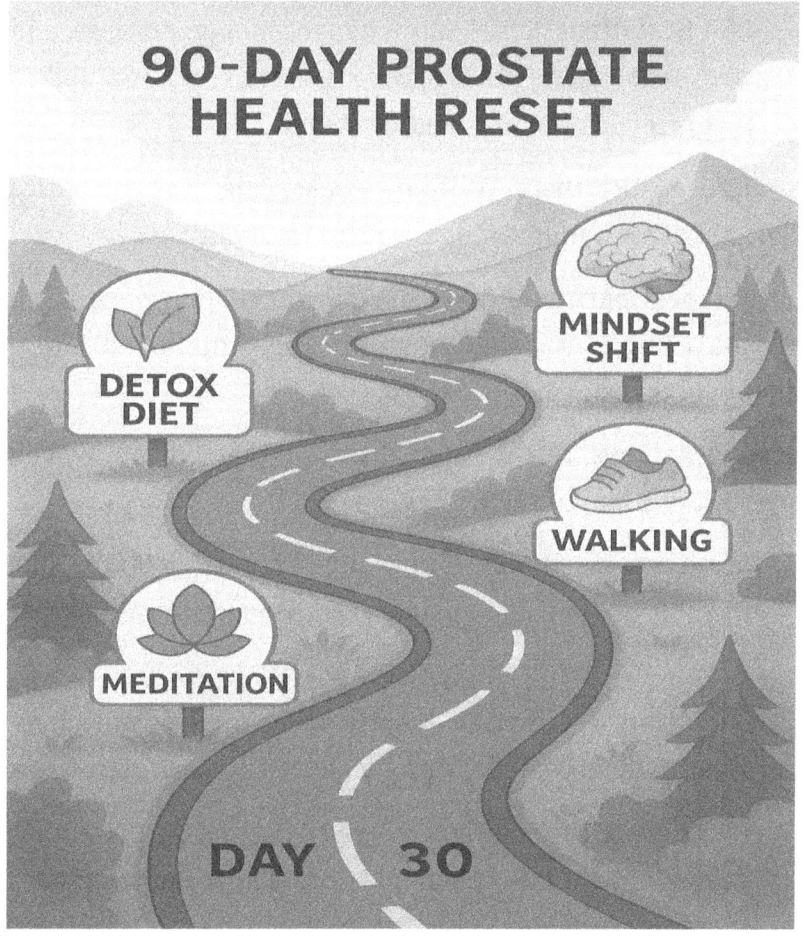

Why 90 days? Because three months is long enough for habits to stick and for biology to respond:

- **Hormones Recalibrate.** Stress hormones, such as cortisol, can decrease with consistent meditation and breathwork. Testosterone balance improves with better sleep and a balanced diet.

- **Inflammation Eases.** Diet changes—like adding tomatoes, green tea, or turmeric—take weeks to lower inflammatory markers that drive prostate cancer progression.

- **PSA Stabilizes.** Small daily changes in diet, exercise, and stress management can prevent those scary PSA spikes that often lead to unnecessary tests.

- **Energy Returns.** Within weeks, men often notice improved stamina, mood, and sleep quality.

Here's the best part: you don't have to do it all at once. Each week, you'll build on small wins until they compound into a fundamental transformation.

This reset follows the *3-Pillar Protocol* that's been woven throughout this book:

1. **Mindset & Stress Control** – Practical tools like meditation, journaling, and breathwork to lower stress and boost resilience.

2. **Nutrition & Lifestyle** – Anti-cancer foods, meal plans, sleep hygiene, and daily movement to nourish your body.

3. **Medical & Integrative Support** – Smarter screening, evidence-based supplements, and safe complementary therapies to strengthen your foundation.

By aligning with these three pillars, the reset works on every level: your mind, your body, and your medical care.

How to Use This Plan?

A plan only works if it feels doable. That's why this reset is structured in weekly steps. Each week you'll add 1–2 simple habits—nothing more. By the end of 13 weeks, you'll have built a complete prostate-protective routine without feeling overwhelmed.

Here's how to use it:

- **One Week at a Time.** Don't jump ahead. Focus on the current week's goals until they feel natural, then move on.
- **Track Your Progress.** Keep a simple journal or use your phone's notes app. Record your sleep quality, energy, mood, and stress. If your doctor orders repeat PSA tests, record those as well.
- **Involve Your Partner or Caregiver.** Having someone walk this journey with you makes it easier to stay accountable and supported. A spouse, friend, or family member can join you in activities such as cooking, walking, or meditation.
- **Be Flexible.** Life happens—miss a day, and that's fine. What matters is consistency over time, not perfection.

Action Step: Before starting, grab a notebook or open a tracking app. Write "Day 1" on the first page. Note how you're currently feeling: energy, mood, sleep, and stress. This will be your baseline—the reference point you'll look back on after 90 days to see how far you've come.

Phase 1: Foundation (Weeks 1–4)

This first month is about laying the groundwork, not overhauling your life overnight. Think of it as setting up scaffolding around your health: you're building a solid structure, one beam at a time. These four weeks focus on getting your breathing, movement, food, and sleep in order—the basics that everything else will build on.

You don't need to rush. In fact, slow and steady is the secret to lasting change. Let's begin.

Week 1: Breathe & Begin

Focus: Stress Reset + Daily Movement

When men hear the word "stress," they often shrug it off as something intangible. But here's the truth: stress is chemistry. Elevated cortisol, the stress hormone, fuels inflammation and worsens PSA variability. Learning to calm your body's "alarm system" is one of the most powerful first steps.

- **Morning Breathwork:** Start each day with 5 minutes of **box breathing**: inhale for 4, hold for 4, exhale for 4, hold for 4. Repeat 6–8 cycles. It's simple, but research shows that even short daily breathwork sessions can reduce cortisol levels and lower blood pressure.

- **Green Tea Swap:** Replace one cup of coffee or soda with green tea. Its catechins are not only antioxidants but have been linked in studies to slowing the progression of prostate cancer.

- **Move Daily:** After each meal, walk for 10 minutes. No stopwatch, no race—just movement. Post-meal walks can improve blood sugar control, aid digestion, and stabilize energy levels.

Action Step: Keep a note on your phone: write down how you feel *before* and *after* breathwork for one week. Many men notice the shift immediately—a sense of calm that lingers through the morning.

Week 2: Food as Medicine

Focus: Add Key Prostate-protective Foods

Now that you've started calming stress, let's feed your body what it craves: fuel that heals. Think of food as your daily prescription.

The Three Food Rules for Week 2:

1. Add **tomatoes** (sauce, paste, or cooked) 3x a week. Lycopene is more bioavailable when cooked.
2. Eat **broccoli or kale** at least 4x this week. Cruciferous vegetables contain sulforaphane, which supports detox pathways.
3. Snack on **walnuts** instead of chips. Rich in omega-3 fatty acids and vitamin E, they support prostate and heart health.

- **Sleep Anchor:** Begin a gentle wind-down routine. Dim lights 30 minutes before bed, set a consistent bedtime, and avoid screens if possible. Quality sleep helps stabilize hormones, strengthens the immune system, and aids in recovery.

Action Step: By the end of the week, write down *one positive shift* you've noticed—better digestion, steadier energy, or even less late-night snacking. Small wins matter.

Week 3: Calm the Mind

Focus: Meditation & Stress Tracking

Your mind is just as important as your body in this reset plan. Anxiety about PSA results or treatment decisions often keeps men in a constant state of fight-or-flight. This week is about reclaiming mental calm.

- **Daily Meditation:** Try *5–10 minutes* of guided meditation each day. Dr. Joe Dispenza's "Blessing of the Energy Centers" is one option, or use a mindfulness app. Studies in cancer patients have shown that meditation reduces cortisol levels, improves sleep quality, and enhances emotional resilience.

- **Track Stress:** Keep a journal of PSA-related anxiety. Write down triggers—like waiting for lab results, or a stressful workday—and what calms you (breathwork, a walk, talking with a partner).

- **Upgrade Movement:** Add **one 20-minute walk** this week. Fresh air and steady movement double as stress relief and cardiovascular training.

Action Step: Each night, write one sentence: *"Today I felt calm when..."* This builds awareness of what actually helps you—your personal stress "medicine."

Week 4: Strengthen the Core

Focus: Pelvic Health + Gentle Yoga

The prostate and pelvic floor work together as a team. Strengthening this region doesn't just improve urinary control—it builds sexual confidence and overall core stability.

- **Pelvic Floor Training (Kegels):** Tighten pelvic muscles as if stopping urination midstream, hold for 5 seconds, release. Do 10 reps, 3 times a day. Over time, this improves urinary control, especially after surgery or treatment.

- **Yoga Intro:** Try two beginner sessions this week. Start with bridge pose (which strengthens the pelvic floor), cat-cow (which improves spinal mobility and provides stress relief), and seated forward bend (which calms the nervous system). Even 15 minutes counts.

- **Track Sleep Quality:** Each morning, rate your sleep 1–10. Notice how breathwork, meditation, and dietary tweaks affect rest.

Action Step: At the end of the week, review your journal. You'll likely notice that your stress, sleep, and energy levels differ from what they were three weeks ago. This reflection reinforces that change is already happening.

End of Month 1 Reflection

You've built a rhythm. You're breathing with intention, eating smarter, walking daily, sleeping deeper, and even strengthening your pelvic floor. None of this required massive willpower—it was about stacking small habits week after week.

Take a moment to look back at your Week 1 notes. Notice how far you've come already. The rest is working, and you've only just begun.

Phase 2: Expansion (Weeks 5–9)

By now, you've built a strong foundation. You're calmer, moving daily, eating smarter, and sleeping better. In Phase 2, we expand those wins into bigger, longer-term changes that strengthen your body, sharpen your mind, and bring your medical care into alignment. Think of this stage as turning a healthy rhythm into momentum.

Week 5: Fuel with Smarter Proteins

Focus: Add Fatty Fish + Reduce Processed Foods

What you eat shapes the inflammation in your body—and inflammation fuels prostate problems. This week, you'll lean on *anti-inflammatory proteins* and trim back the culprits.

- **Add 2 servings of fatty fish:** Salmon, sardines, or mackerel twice this week. Omega-3 fatty acids calm inflammation and support cardiovascular and prostate health.

- **Cut back processed meats:** Swap bacon, sausages, and deli meats for grilled chicken, beans, or tofu. These foods are linked to a higher risk of cancer.

- **Tame sugar spikes:** Choose fruit over pastries, and water or green tea over soda. Stable blood sugar helps lower cancer-driving inflammation.

Action Step: Write down your protein choices for each meal this week. Notice how swapping bacon for salmon, or chips for walnuts, changes your energy and digestion.

Week 6: Build Strength, Build Resilience

Focus: Introduce Strength Training

Muscle isn't just for athletes—it's medicine for all. More lean muscle improves insulin sensitivity, lowers inflammation, and helps regulate hormones that influence prostate cancer progression.

- **2 strength sessions per week:** Start simple with bodyweight moves—pushups, squats, lunges, and planks. If you prefer, use light dumbbells or resistance bands.
- **Keep it short:** Even 20 minutes twice a week can improve strength, balance, and confidence.
- **Pelvic reinforcement:** Continue Kegels—pair them with core work for added bladder control.

Action Step: Schedule two strength sessions in your calendar this week. Treat them like doctor's appointments: non-negotiable.

Week 7: Medical Check-In & Vitamin D

Focus: Review Progress + Test Under Control

This reset isn't just about lifestyle—it's also about smart medical choices. By week 7, it's time to check in with your doctor.

- **Repeat PSA test:** If your doctor agrees, request a PSA under controlled conditions (no sex or cycling 48 hours before). This ensures accurate results and avoids false scares.

- **Ask for vitamin D:** A blood test can reveal deficiency, which is common in men and linked to worse prostate outcomes. If low, supplement (often 2,000 IU daily, but confirm dose with your doctor).

- **Bring your journal:** Show your provider your notes on diet, sleep, and stress. It gives them context beyond the numbers.

Action Step: Book your appointment. Write down 3 questions you'll ask—such as *"What's my PSA velocity?"* or *"Should I consider supplements?"*

Week 8: Flow with Tai Chi or Qigong

Focus: Gentle Movement for Balance and Calm

This week, you'll add a practice that has stood the test of time—literally thousands of years. *Tai Chi* and *Qigong* combine gentle movement, breathwork, and focus to reduce stress and boost circulation.

- **Daily 15 minutes:** Follow a beginner video online or join a local class. Movements are slow, flowing, and easy to learn.

- **Proven benefits:** Studies in cancer survivors show Tai Chi reduces stress, improves immunity, and even enhances sleep quality.

- **Mind-body bridge:** This is meditation in motion, blending mindfulness with physical strength.

Action Step: Choose a 10–15-minute routine (YouTube, app, or DVD). Practice every morning or evening, then journal how calm or energized you feel afterward.

Week 9: Smart Supplement Integration

Focus: Add Evidence-based Supplements

Not all supplements are effective, but some are supported by research when used wisely and under medical supervision. This week is about layering in support—without falling for hype.

- **Beta-Sitosterol:** Shown to improve urinary flow and reduce frequency, especially in men with enlarged prostates.
- **Zinc:** Essential for prostate function and hormone regulation; deficiency is common in aging men.
- **Vitamin D:** If you tested low in Week 7, continue supplementation as prescribed.

Important: Always consult with your oncologist or doctor before taking supplements. Some can interact with medications or treatments.

Action Step: Make a supplement list (include brand, dose, and timing). Share it with your doctor for approval before starting.

End of Month 2 Reflection

You've expanded your reset to include smarter food swaps, strength training, regular medical check-ins, calming Tai Chi, and targeted supplements. At this point, your body should feel stronger, your stress should be more manageable, and your plan should be more sustainable. The pieces are coming together—you're not just reacting to prostate cancer; you're actively reshaping your health.

Phase 3: Integration (Weeks 10–13)

You've built the foundation, expanded your habits, and now it's time for integration. These final four weeks are about cementing routines into your life so they're not just a "program," but part of your identity. Think of this phase as **practice for the rest of your life**—a chance to test what works, fine-tune your approach, and create your own prostate-protective lifestyle.

Week 10: Healing Touch

Focus: Acupuncture or Massage for Stress and Relief

By now, you've tackled breathwork, meditation, and movement—but physical therapies can also play a powerful role in calming the nervous system and easing treatment side effects.

- **Acupuncture:** Proven in cancer care to reduce fatigue, improve sleep, and ease hot flashes and urinary discomfort. Sessions typically last 30–60 minutes, costing between $50 and $100, and some insurance plans cover them.
- **Massage:** Helps relax muscles, reduce anxiety, and improve circulation. Even a 30-minute session can leave you calmer and less tense.

Action Step: Book one session this week—either acupuncture or massage—and track your feelings for 24 hours afterward. Write down changes in pain, stress, or sleep.

Week 11: Spice & Simplify

Focus: Daily Turmeric + Reduce Alcohol and Sugar

Nutrition is a marathon, not a sprint. This week, you'll refine the anti-cancer diet by focusing on two key moves.

- **Add Turmeric + Black Pepper Daily:** Just ½ teaspoon of turmeric with a pinch of black pepper in food or tea boosts curcumin absorption. Curcumin has been studied for its anti-inflammatory and anticancer properties, particularly in relation to prostate health.
- **Cut Back Alcohol and Sugary Drinks:** Even modest alcohol intake can fuel inflammation. Replacing that evening beer with sparkling water and lime, or soda with green tea, helps lower risk factors.

Action Step: Choose one meal each day to add turmeric + pepper. At the same time, cut at least one sugary or alcoholic drink from your week. Write down the swaps you made.

Week 12: Track & Reflect

Focus: Monitor Progress in Key Areas

Before you graduate from this reset, it's time to measure your wins. Don't just rely on numbers like PSA—look at your whole life.

- **Journal check-in:** Record how your energy, sleep, stress, mood, and urinary function compare to Week 1.
- **Partner perspective:** Ask your partner or caregiver what changes they've noticed. Sometimes others see progress before we do.
- **Celebrate non-scale victories:** Better sleep, calmer mornings, less worry, or feeling more in control.

Action Step: Write a one-page *"reset reflection."* Note your biggest wins, what surprised you, and what still feels challenging.

Week 13: Build Your Forever Plan

Focus: Keep What Works, Let Go of What Doesn't

The *90-Day Reset* ends here, but your new life begins. The final step is choosing which habits to keep long-term.

- **Select your core 5:** Circle the five habits you'll keep forever (e.g., daily breathwork, two fish meals weekly, yoga, supplements, turmeric).
- **Set your medical rhythm:** Plan your next PSA test and doctor visit—this keeps momentum and accountability.
- **Celebrate:** Mark the milestone with something meaningful—a walk with family, a special meal, or even sharing your progress with your support group.

Action Step: Write down your *Forever Plan*—a simple 1-page list of your ongoing habits. Keep it visible on your fridge, mirror, or journal as a daily reminder that you've built a healthier, stronger version of yourself.

End of Month 3 Reflection

You've done it. Ninety days ago, this was just a plan on paper. Now, it's your life. You've lowered stress, cleaned up your diet, moved your body, and built new rhythms that support healing. Even if your PSA hasn't dropped dramatically yet, you've created the environment where healing can happen.

This reset isn't the end. It's your launchpad. The man who once felt overwhelmed by too many changes is now living proof: step by step, you can reclaim your health, one habit at a time.

Measuring Progress

One of the most empowering parts of the 90-Day Reset is seeing your progress unfold. But here's the secret: progress isn't just about numbers on a lab report. It's about how you *feel*—in your body, in your mind, and in your daily life.

What to Track?

- **PSA levels:** If your doctor recommends testing during or after the reset, note your result—and just as important, whether it's stable or rising slowly. Remember: PSA is a clue, not a verdict.

- **Urinary function:** Keep a simple log. Are you waking up fewer times at night? Is your flow stronger? Are you using fewer pads or none at all?

- **Energy:** Rate your energy from 1–10 each day. Do mornings feel lighter? Can you walk further without feeling fatigued?

- **Sleep:** Track bedtime, wake time, and sleep quality. Even one extra hour of deep sleep can transform your recovery.

- **Mood:** Note your stress, anxiety, or calmness. A short line in your journal—*"Felt calm during meditation"* or *"Less anxious about results"*—is enough.

Psychological Markers

Progress isn't only physical. A successful reset also brings:

- **Reduced anxiety:** You don't wake up in a panic about your next PSA.

- **Improved confidence:** You feel more in control of your health and choices.

- **Resilience:** You bounce back faster from stress or setbacks.

Action Step: Use a simple journal or a note-taking app on your phone. At the end of each week, jot down: *"What improved? What still feels hard? What am I proud of?"* Over time, you'll see a clear trajectory toward better health and peace of mind.

Case Example — David's Reset Journey

David, a 62-year-old teacher, came to me after his PSA had climbed to 6.2. He was tired, 25 pounds overweight, and anxious about intimacy—urinary leakage and fatigue were holding him back. "I feel like my body is betraying me," he admitted during our first conversation.

Instead of throwing everything at him at once, we put him on the *90-Day Reset*, one step at a time.

- In **Month 1**, he started with breathwork, daily walks, and swapping soda for green tea. His sleep improved within two weeks, and he felt calmer.

- In **Month 2**, he added fish twice a week, strength training, and meditation. By week 8, he had lost 12 pounds and noticed stronger bladder control.

- In **Month 3**, he layered in turmeric, cut back alcohol, and tried Tai Chi. By week 13, his PSA had stabilized at 6.1—no further rise—and he had lost 20 pounds in total. Most importantly, he told me, "My wife and I feel close again. Intimacy isn't something I dread anymore."

David's story mirrors what research shows: a steady, structured reset doesn't just change lab numbers—it transforms quality of life.

Action Step: As you follow the reset, picture your own *"David moment."* What does success look like for you—fewer bathroom trips? Better energy? More confidence with your partner? Write it down now. That vision will keep you motivated when change feels slow.

Key Takeaway

Morning rituals such as green tea meditation, a turmeric smoothie, and gentle stretching are quick, inexpensive, and supported by research. Together, they build confidence, resilience, and a healthier daily rhythm.

Key Takeaways

- **Small steps create big change.** You don't need to overhaul your life in a day. Layering just 1–2 new habits each week helps build momentum without feeling overwhelmed.

- **The three pillars matter most.** Mindset & stress control, nutrition & lifestyle, and medical & integrative support work together like gears—when one moves, the others follow.

- **Consistency beats perfection.** Daily walks, green tea, meditation, and prostate-protective foods are most potent when practiced regularly, even if imperfectly.

- **Integrate, don't replace.** Complementary therapies—such as yoga, acupuncture, and targeted supplements—work best when added to standard care, rather than used in place of it.

- **The reset builds resilience.** Within 90 days, men often report lower stress, stronger intimacy, stabilized PSA, and renewed hope for the future.

- **The "Forever Plan" is the real goal.** The reset is a launchpad. The habits you choose to carry forward—whether breathwork, diet shifts, or weekly movement—are the ones that protect your prostate for life.

CHAPTER 8
THE LONGEVITY PROTOCOL

"Fall seven times and stand up eight."
— *Japanese Proverb*

Imagine this: you've made it through diagnosis, endured treatment, and finally stepped into survivorship. Friends and family call you a fighter. Doctors nod with approval. Life is supposed to go back to *"normal."*

But then it happens—your calendar reminder pops up: *PSA test this week.* Your chest tightens. You sit in the waiting room, staring at the lab slip, every second dragging. The thought runs like a ticker tape in your mind: *Will the number stay steady… or creep up?*

You're not alone. More than *3.5 million men in the U.S.* are living with a history of prostate cancer as of 2025, and almost all of them know the weight of this question.[71] Each test feels like a verdict—sometimes more stressful than the treatment itself. Survivorship brings relief, yes, but also a new challenge: how to keep cancer from coming back, and how to live fully without letting fear ruin your life.

Here's the truth: *recurrence is not inevitable.* In fact, research shows that the right lifestyle changes after treatment can lower the risk of cancer-specific mortality and recurrence by *20–30%.* That's not a small number—it's a game changer.[72]

And this is where the idea of a *longevity protocol* comes in. Think of it as your personal blueprint for staying healthy:

- **Three essential medical tests** to track your progress.
- **Four daily habits** to strengthen your resilience.
- **Five caregiver strategies** that turn survivorship into a team effort.

This is not about perfection. It's not about overhauling your life overnight. It's about building a steady, science-backed rhythm that keeps you strong and confident.

So, let me reassure you: **survival isn't the finish line—it's the beginning of a new chapter.** One where you're not just avoiding recurrence, but actively building a healthier, longer, and fuller life.

In this chapter, I'll show you exactly how to do it—how to track the right markers, weave protective habits into your days, and lean on the people who want to see you thrive. You'll also meet a survivor who turned vigilance into victory, proving that the fear of recurrence doesn't have to define you.

Three Medical Checkpoints

When treatment ends, many men want to slam the door shut on hospitals and lab tests. But here's the reality: the follow-up phase is just as important as the treatment itself. About *20–30%* of men experience recurrence within ten years, and catching it early often means the difference between a quick course of targeted therapy versus more aggressive treatment down the road.[73]

Think of these three checkpoints—PSA monitoring, imaging when indicated, and advanced blood tests like *circulating tumor cells (CTCs)*—as your personal radar system. Each one scans the horizon in its own way, giving you an early warning if trouble is brewing.

TESTS FOR PROSTATE CANCER

PSA Test
☐ Date: _____

Positron Emission Tomography (PET) Scan
☐ Date: _____

Circulating Tumor Cells (CTCs) Testing
☐ Date: _____

1. PSA Monitoring: More Than Just a Number

PSA is still the gold standard of prostate cancer follow-up. After surgery, your PSA should drop to undetectable levels (usually below 0.1 ng/mL). After radiation, it may not hit zero, but the trend should be steadily downward.

What matters most is not a single reading—it's the velocity (how fast PSA rises) and the doubling time (how quickly it multiplies). For example:

- A rise of *0.2 ng/mL* within six months is a red flag.[74]

- A PSA doubling time under 12 months also signals a higher risk of recurrence.

Action Step: Test every 3–6 months for the first five years, then annually if the condition remains stable. Keep a PSA journal—record not only the values and dates, but also how you felt at each test. Many men find that tracking both numbers and emotions helps them manage anxiety.

2. Imaging When Indicated: The Power of PSMA PET

If PSA begins to creep up, it's time to ask: *Where is the cancer hiding?* That's where imaging comes in. Standard CT or bone scans often miss small or early metastases. However, the game changer in recent years has been the *PSMA PET scan*.

PSMA PET uses a special tracer that latches onto prostate cancer cells, lighting them up like a beacon. Studies show that it detects recurrence with approximately *90% accuracy*—even when the PSA level is as low as *0.5 ng/mL*.[75] That means doctors can find and zap tiny lesions long before they spread widely.

Costs vary ($2,000–$4,000, depending on insurance), but the precision it offers can help avoid unnecessary systemic treatments.

Action Step: Don't rush to scan at every PSA bump. Instead, ask your doctor:

- *"When would imaging be necessary for me?"*
- *"Is PSMA PET the best choice in my case, or is MRI enough?"*

This ensures you get the right scan at the right time—not too much, not too little.

3. Circulating Tumor Cells (CTCs): The Liquid Biopsy of the Future

Imagine finding traces of cancer activity with just a blood test. That's the promise of *CTC testing*. Known as a *"liquid biopsy,"* it looks for prostate cancer cells drifting in the bloodstream.

Right now, it's still more common in research centers, though one method (CellSearch) is FDA-approved for advanced prostate cancer. In follow-up care, it's not yet routine, but it can sometimes detect recurrence earlier than PSA or imaging alone.

Studies show CTCs are found in *10–30% of men* with higher-risk disease.[76] That means the test is not perfect, but when used alongside PSA and scans, it may soon become part of standard survivorship care.

A Story of Vigilance Paying Off

Take *Mark*, a 62-year-old retired mechanic. After his surgery, he kept up with quarterly PSA tests. For a while, numbers stayed flat. Then one test came back at *0.3 ng/mL*—still low, but higher than it should have been. His oncologist ordered a PSMA PET scan, which revealed a single, tiny lesion that was invisible on regular imaging. With targeted radiation, Mark avoided more invasive therapy.

As he told me later, *"Those tests saved me. If I had waited, I'd be in a much tougher fight right now."*

Important Note

These three checkpoints—PSA monitoring, smart use of imaging, and emerging tools like CTCs—form the backbone of your longevity plan. They don't just measure numbers; they give you **time, options, and control.**

Four Lifestyle Changes to Block Recurrence

When the hospital visits slow down and the treatment is behind you, the big question often becomes: *"What now?"* For many men, the fear of recurrence lingers like a shadow. Here's the good news: you don't need to overhaul your entire life to stack the odds in your favor. Small, repeatable daily habits can lower inflammation, steady your hormones, and strengthen your body's natural defenses against prostate cancer.

Think of it as building armor one piece at a time. Research shows that simple lifestyle changes can reduce cancer-specific mortality and recurrence risk by *20–30%*.[77] That's not theory—that's science in action. Here are four core habits every survivor can use to build resilience.

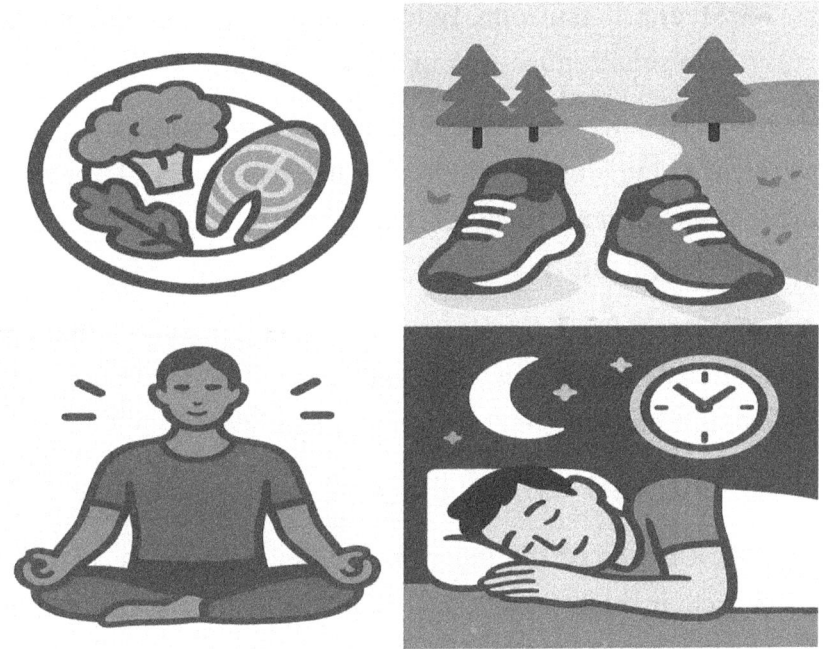

CORE LONGEVITY HABITS

1. Regular Exercise

Your body was designed to move, and staying active after treatment does more than just keep weight off—it lowers inflammation, boosts immune function, and helps regulate testosterone levels. Studies consistently show that men who exercise regularly have lower recurrence rates and live longer.[78]

Here's the formula:

- **150 minutes of moderate activity** per week (brisk walking, swimming, or cycling).

- **Strength training twice weekly** (bodyweight moves like squats, push-ups, or light weights).

One survivor I worked with, a 59-year-old teacher, set a goal of simply walking for 15 minutes after lunch every day. Over time, those walks became longer, his weight dropped by 10 pounds, and his energy returned.

Action Step: Print a calendar and tick off every day you complete 20+ minutes of movement. Seeing the streak build can be just as motivating as the exercise itself.

2. The Anti-Cancer Plate

Your fork is one of the most potent tools against recurrence. Diets rich in plant-forward, anti-inflammatory foods reduce cancer-promoting pathways. On the flip side, excess sugar, alcohol, and processed meats stoke inflammation.

- **Eat more of:** Cooked tomatoes, cruciferous vegetables (broccoli, kale, Brussels sprouts), turmeric with black pepper, fatty fish (salmon, sardines), soy foods, pomegranate, and nuts.
- **Cut back on:** Processed meats (bacon, deli meats), sugary drinks, and alcohol beyond moderation.

Action Step: On Sunday, prep one batch of *"anti-cancer"* meals for the week—think a pot of tomato-broccoli lentil soup, a tray of turmeric-roasted salmon, or pomegranate-topped quinoa bowls.

3. No Smoking

Smoking is a well-established risk factor for worse outcomes after prostate cancer. A population-based study of men aged 40–

64 found that those who smoked at the time of diagnosis had more than twice the risk of prostate cancer-specific mortality compared with men who never smoked.[79] This higher risk remained significant even after accounting for tumor stage, Gleason score, and primary treatment, showing that smoking itself can directly influence long-term prognosis.

Action Step: If you smoke, make this the week you take your first step toward quitting. Call the free national Quitline (1-800-QUIT-NOW), download a quit-smoking app, or talk to your doctor about nicotine replacement options. Every cigarette avoided lowers your risk and strengthens your recovery.

3. Better Sleep

Sleep isn't passive—it's when your body repairs, balances hormones, and restores immune strength. Poor sleep has been linked to a higher risk of aggressive prostate cancer.[80]

- **Target:** 7–8 hours of high-quality sleep per night.
- **Bedtime Ritual:** Dim lights 30 minutes before bed, avoid screens, and try gentle stretches or breathing.
- **Digital Sunset:** Create a hard stop on devices—no screens 30 minutes before bed.

Action Step: Rate your sleep quality each morning on a scale of 1–10. Watch how it improves as you stick with breathwork, meditation, and nutrition shifts.

4. Mindset & Stress Reset

Your mind can be your greatest ally—or your biggest saboteur. Stress isn't just an emotion; it drives inflammation, disrupts hormones, and weakens immune defenses. Chronic stress has been linked with higher PSA and worse cancer outcomes.

- **Meditation & Breathwork:** Meditation or breathwork for *10 minutes a day* lowers cortisol.[81] Dr. Joe Dispenza's guided practices or simple mindfulness apps can help rewire stress patterns.

- **Journaling:** Tracking triggers—like PSA anxiety or sleepless nights—helps you see patterns and take control.

Action Step: Start (or end) each day with 10 minutes of guided meditation. Follow it by jotting down one line in your journal: *"Today I felt calm when..."* It's simple, but it rewires how your brain perceives stress.

A Survivor's Note

One of my patients, a 68-year-old grandfather, committed to these habits after finishing radiation. He lost 12 pounds, slept better than he had in years, and began journaling nightly. *"I feel stronger,"* he told me, *"and my PSA is undetectable."* His story proves the point: resilience isn't built in a hospital; it's built through the small, daily choices you make at home.

> **Remember**
> These five habits—moving your body, eating smart, staying smoke-free, calming your mind, and protecting your sleep—aren't flashy, but they're life-changing. Done consistently, they build resilience, lower your risk of recurrence, and give you back not just more years, but better years.

Caregiver & Support Strategies

A prostate cancer journey never belongs to just one person—it inevitably ripples through families, partners, and close friends. Survivors often carry physical and emotional weight, but caregivers shoulder a unique burden too: they become advocates, organizers, cheerleaders, and anchors when fear or fatigue sets in.

TOP 5 TIPS
FOR CAREGIVERS

1. Track Appointments and Tests

 2. Cook Anti-Cancer Meals

3. Encourage and Join Exercise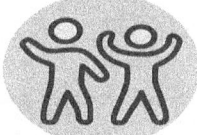

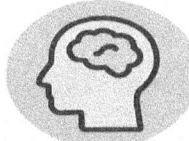 4. Watch for Mental Health Changes

5. Practice Stress Relief Together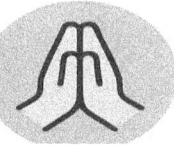

The good news? Research consistently shows that when caregivers are actively engaged—whether attending appointments, cooking healthier meals, or simply listening—

men are more likely to adhere to treatment plans, recover more quickly, and feel emotionally supported. Caregiving, at its best, isn't about doing everything *for* someone—it's about doing life *with* them.

Here are five practical strategies that transform caregiving from a source of stress into a shared path of resilience.

1. Shared Vigilance

Fear of recurrence can feel like a cloud hanging over every PSA test. Caregivers can play a pivotal role in lifting that weight by becoming part of the monitoring process. Attending appointments, writing down questions, and noting the doctor's answers provide not only clarity but also reassurance that nothing slips through the cracks.

Action Step: Keep a joint *"health notebook."* Record every test, PSA value, and doctor's explanation. Add space for your own reflections—how you both felt before and after each visit. Over time, this notebook becomes a record of progress and a reminder that you're navigating the journey together.

2. Emotional Anchoring

PSA anxiety is real, and it affects both the man being tested and the person sitting beside him. Waiting for results can stir sleepless nights, irritability, or a sense of dread. Research shows that about one in five prostate cancer survivors experience clinical depression.[82] Caregivers can help by creating rituals that steady emotions during these high-stress times.

One couple I worked with took a quiet walk to their favorite park before every lab draw. "It gave us a sense of control," the wife said, "and helped us face the day together."

Action Step: Build a *"calm-before-test"* ritual—whether it's prayer, yoga stretches, a shared meditation, or even a favorite playlist on the car ride. These anchors not only ease stress but also transform the test day into a shared moment of strength.

3. Nutrition Partnership

Food choices are easier—and far more sustainable—when they're made together. Men who try to overhaul their diet in isolation often feel deprived, but when caregivers join in, it becomes a shared lifestyle rather than a restriction.

Cooking prostate-protective meals—such as tomato soups, turmeric-spiced salmon, broccoli stir-fries, or pomegranate smoothies—benefits both partners. It's not just about nutrients; it's about building a rhythm of health in the home.

Action Step: Create a joint grocery list once a week. Include three *"must-have"* anti-cancer foods and plan two meals you'll both enjoy. Cooking and eating together shift the focus from sacrifice to connection.

4. Encourage and Join Exercise

Exercise adherence nearly doubles when it's done with a partner. Whether it's a brisk evening walk, a gentle yoga class, or even dancing in the living room, moving together makes activity less of a chore and more of a shared experience.

One caregiver told me, *"Our daily walks were as much for my sanity as his."* Science backs her up: movement lowers stress, reduces inflammation, and improves the mental health of both partners. Research also shows that men who exercise regularly after prostate cancer treatment have a lower risk of recurrence and improved overall survival.[83]

Action Step: Choose one activity you both enjoy—such as walking, tai chi, or a weekly dance session—and schedule it like an appointment. Protect this time as fiercely as you would have a medical check-up.

5. Celebrating Milestones

Living with vigilance doesn't mean life has to feel clinical. Marking progress—whether it's a stable PSA, an anniversary of treatment completion, or sticking with a 30-day diet plan—creates moments of joy that carry both patient and caregiver through the tougher days.

One family I worked with celebrated every stable PSA with a special dinner where everyone named one thing they were grateful for. "It reminded us that life was still ours," the son said.

Action Step: Create small rituals to celebrate wins—such as dinner out, a gratitude journal entry, or a family event. These celebrations keep motivation alive and transform medical milestones into life milestones.

The Caregiver's Power

Caregivers are more than companions; they are co-pilots on this journey of longevity. Through shared vigilance, emotional anchoring, nutrition support, movement, and celebration, they turn fear into teamwork and routine into ritual.

If you are a caregiver reading this, know this: your presence, encouragement, and steady hand are as powerful as any prescription. Together, you and your loved one can write a future defined not by recurrence-anxiety but by resilience, connection, and hope.

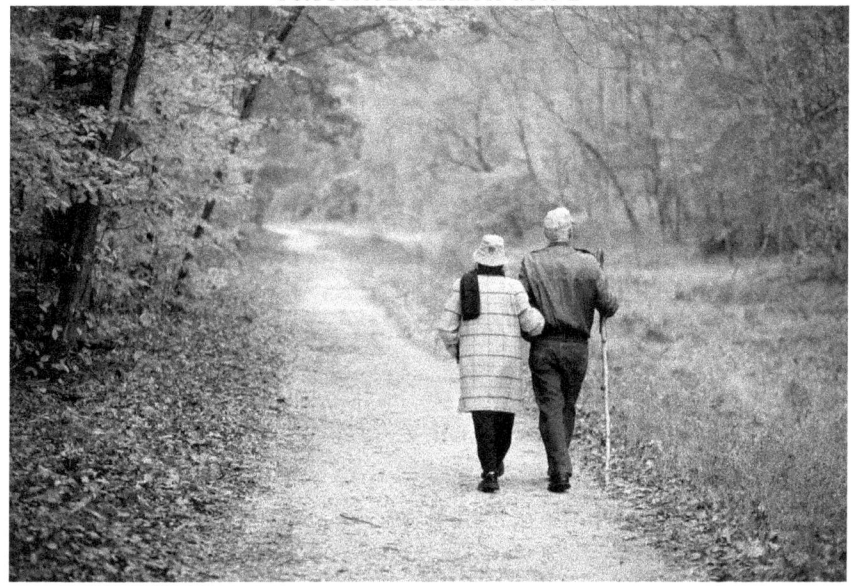

Case Study

Mark, a 63-year-old executive, thought his prostate cancer journey had ended in 2019 after a successful prostatectomy. For two years, his PSA remained undetectable. Then came the call no survivor wants: his PSA had crept up to 0.4 ng/mL. Fear of recurrence resurfaced. Instead of panicking, Mark decided to take control with a step-by-step longevity protocol.

He began by overhauling his daily routine. He lost 15 pounds by shifting to a mostly plant-based diet built around kale salads, tomato-based soups, tofu stir-fries, and salmon twice a week. He quit smoking after two decades, replaced late-night emails with eight hours of sleep, and started a morning meditation practice to tame stress. Every three months, he logged his PSA results in a journal—not just the number, but also how he felt before and after each test.

When his PSA nudged up again to 0.5 ng/mL, his oncologist recommended a PSMA PET scan. The scan detected a small pelvic node that older imaging would have likely missed. Thanks to this early detection, targeted radiation successfully eliminated the lesion, and within 18 months, his PSA level had returned to undetectable levels. Follow-up scans showed no sign of disease.

Mark's wife was an equal partner in his *reset*. She joined him on daily walks, cooked anti-cancer meals alongside him, and even practiced yoga together on weekends. "We tackled it together," Mark said. "I felt stronger knowing I wasn't doing it alone."

The results went beyond his lab numbers. He reported feeling calmer, more energetic, and even noticed an improvement in intimacy—proof that quality of life can rebound alongside medical progress.

Mark's story highlights a simple but powerful truth: longevity isn't luck, it's built. His success came not from one "miracle cure," but from stacking small, consistent habits—diet, exercise, stress control, sleep—alongside vigilant medical monitoring and caregiver support.

Lesson: By combining three checkpoints (PSA, PET scans, CTCs), four daily habits (movement, anti-cancer nutrition, stress reset, restorative sleep), and active caregiver involvement, survivors can transform vigilance into victory.

Mark's journey shows that survivorship is not passive. It's a lifelong protocol—a shield of habits, tests, and support that keeps recurrence at bay.

Key Takeaways

- **Vigilance is protection.** A structured longevity protocol—regular monitoring, lifestyle changes, and caregiver support—can lower recurrence risk by 20–30%.

- **Trust the three checkpoints.** PSA velocity, PSMA PET imaging, and circulating tumor cell (CTC) tests are your strongest tools for catching recurrence early.

- **Follow a clear rhythm.** PSA every 3–6 months for the first two years, then annually if stable. Any rise or rapid doubling time deserves immediate follow-up.

- **Stack daily habits.** Weight control, quitting smoking, restorative sleep, and stress management can all help reduce inflammation, balance hormones, and strengthen immunity.

- **Make it a team effort.** Caregivers amplify success through shared calendars, meal prep, exercise routines, emotional check-ins, and stress-relief practices.

- **Measure and adapt.** Use journals or apps to track PSA values, mood, energy, and lifestyle habits. If PSA trends shift, discuss advanced imaging or CTC testing with your doctor.

CHAPTER 9
THRIVING BEYOND CANCER

"Although the world is full of suffering, it is also full of the overcoming of it."
— Helen Keller

When David rang the bell at his cancer center to mark the end of radiation, he expected to feel only relief. Instead, he walked out the doors with gnawing emptiness. His doctors had cleared him, his PSA looked good, but he whispered to his wife on the drive home, *"Now what? Who am I if I'm not fighting cancer anymore?"*

That quiet question is one many men wrestle with. Treatment may end, but survivorship brings its own set of challenges: the lingering fear of recurrence, changes in intimacy, shifts in identity, and the pressure to *"bounce back"* when your body and emotions are still adjusting. The truth? Surviving prostate cancer isn't the finish line—it's the starting line of a new chapter you get to design.

Thriving beyond cancer is not about pretending it never happened. It's about rewriting your story so that the scars become symbols of resilience, not reminders of loss. Research backs this up: studies show men who engage in intentional survivorship practices—whether through mindset work, lifestyle changes, or community involvement—report higher quality of life, less anxiety, and deeper relationships compared to those who *"just move on."*

This chapter is your map for that new life. You'll learn:

- **Three mindset shifts** that can help transform fear into focus and loss into purpose.
- **Five intimacy tools** to restore connection and confidence in your relationship.
- **Three ways to give back** so that your experience becomes fuel for helping others.
- And a **case study of one survivor** who discovered not just how to live again, but how to live better.

The point is simple: you don't have to settle for merely surviving. With the right tools and perspective, you can thrive—mentally, physically, and emotionally. Let's start by reimagining what life after cancer can look like.

Three Mindset Shifts

Recovery after prostate cancer isn't only about PSA numbers, medical tests, or even diet. It's also about the story you tell yourself each day. For many men, survivorship brings invisible struggles—fear of recurrence, depression, and a loss of identity. But here's the good news: with the right mindset, you can rewrite the story. You're not just surviving—you're building a new life.

Below are three powerful shifts that research, patient stories, and clinical practice all show can make the difference between living in fear and thriving with purpose.

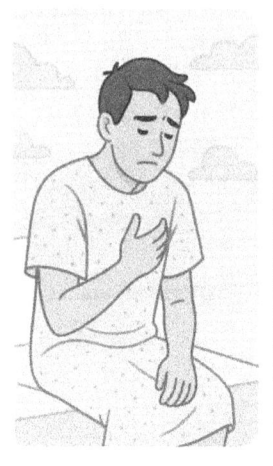 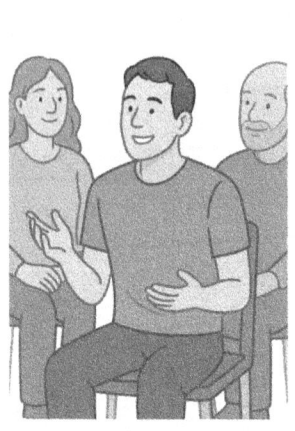 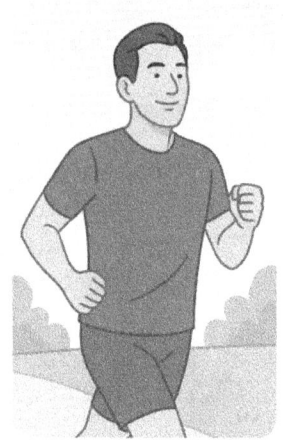

1. ANXIOUS   2. LEARNING   3. GROWTH

1. From Fear to Focus

Fear of recurrence is real. Studies suggest up to 87% of survivors experience it at some point.[84] But fear doesn't have to be the driver of your life—it can be redirected into fuel.

Instead of obsessing over every PSA result, shift your focus to what you can actually control: **your daily actions**. Sleep. Movement. Diet. Stress. Each of these is within your grasp and has real, measurable effects on your health.

Take Tom, a 58-year-old survivor who once described his anxiety before every blood test as "a punch in the gut." Instead of trying to push the fear away, he began using it as a signal to double down on healthy routines: morning walks, swapping soda for green tea, and sticking to a bedtime schedule. *"Now every PSA feels like a report card on my habits, not just my cancer,"* he told me.

Action Step: Journal one daily win that has nothing to do with cancer. A walk, a laugh with a friend, a meal you're proud of. Over time, these notes will remind you that your life is bigger than a lab result.

2. From Isolation to Connection

Prostate cancer can be lonely. Symptoms like incontinence, fatigue, or intimacy challenges can make men withdraw, feeling ashamed or *"different."* But silence only magnifies the weight.

Research shows that survivors who join peer groups or involve caregivers experience lower anxiety, greater resilience, and stronger follow-through on treatment plans.[85] Even a single supportive conversation can help reframe the journey.

Take James, a 62-year-old retiree who initially kept everything bottled up. When his wife encouraged him to attend a local support group, he reluctantly went—only to find half the room shared his same fears. *"I thought I was broken,"* he admitted. *"Turns out, I was just human."*

Action Step: Join one support circle this month—online, through your local cancer center, or in your community. If that feels daunting, start smaller: share one worry with a trusted friend or partner. Each act of openness chips away at the wall of isolation.

3. From Loss to Purpose

Many survivors feel diminished—physically, emotionally, even professionally. The cancer may be behind them, but it sometimes leaves scars on confidence, intimacy, and self-image. The key is reframing this loss into a new purpose.

Studies show men who find meaning—whether through mentoring, volunteering, or creative pursuits—report a higher quality of life and less depression. Purpose is not about going back to *"who you were before cancer."* It's about discovering who you can become now.

One patient, Daniel, a former business executive, struggled with identity after retiring early due to treatment side effects. Over time, he began volunteering at a local hospital, where he spoke with newly diagnosed men. *"I lost my old job,"* he said, *"but I gained a calling."* His new purpose gave him back the dignity and confidence he feared were gone forever.

Action Step: Write down three things cancer has taught you that you want to carry forward—whether it's gratitude, resilience, or a new perspective on relationships. Let these guideposts shape your *"after-cancer"* life.

Bottom Line

These three shifts—fear into focus, isolation into connection, and loss into purpose—are the mental foundation for thriving beyond prostate cancer. Your body has healed; now it's time for your mind to follow suit.

Intimacy Tips for Couples

Prostate cancer changes more than lab values and treatment schedules—it often reshapes how couples experience closeness. Surgeries, radiation, or hormone therapies can affect sexual function, body confidence, and relationship dynamics. Research shows nearly half of all survivors face erectile dysfunction, and many couples report increased strain in their emotional and physical connection during recovery.[86] Yet here's the truth: intimacy is not defined by performance alone. It's about connection, creativity, and communication.

The good news? Many couples emerge stronger when they approach intimacy as a shared journey, not a problem to fix.

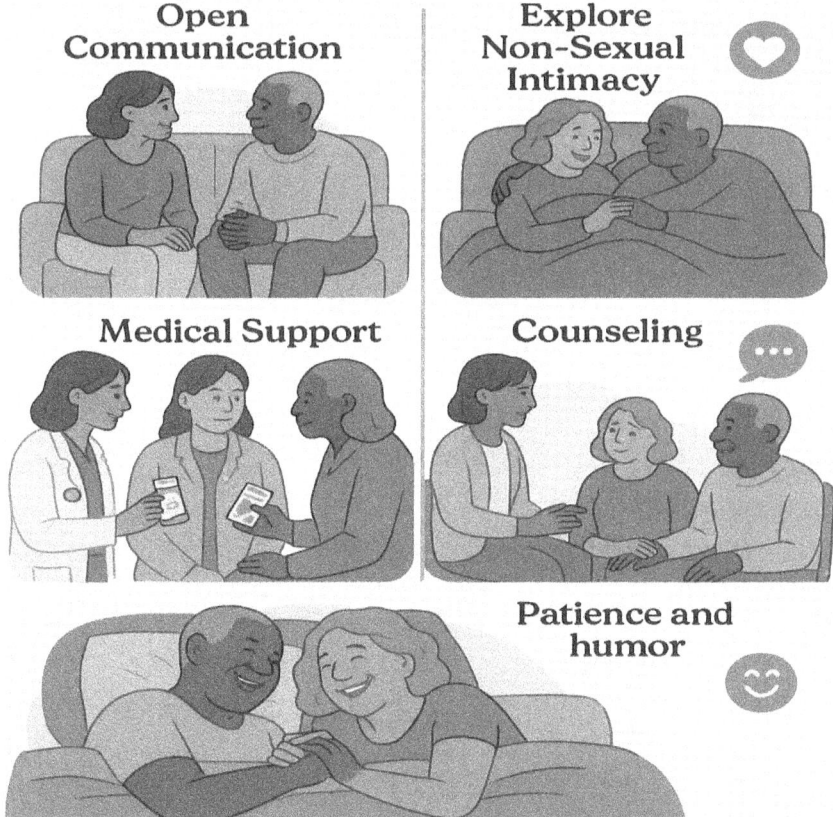

Here are five evidence-based, practical strategies to help you and your partner rediscover closeness.

1. Open Communication: Say the Unsaid

The most powerful intimacy tool isn't medication or technique—it's conversation. Silence breeds shame, but speaking honestly creates space for healing. Couples who talk openly about fears, desires, and frustrations often report stronger satisfaction and less anxiety.

Instead of waiting for the *"perfect moment,"* start gently. Try: *"I want us to feel close. Can we explore what works for us now?"* These talks are not just about erections—they're about understanding each other's evolving needs and adjusting expectations together.

Action Step: End each day by asking your partner one question: *"What made you feel connected today?"* Even a two-minute exchange can build trust.

2. Redefine Intimacy: Beyond Performance

Intimacy is bigger than sex—it's the daily rituals of touch, affection, and presence. Holding hands, a warm bath together, a back rub, or cuddling on the couch all trigger oxytocin, the bonding hormone that fosters closeness.

One couple I worked with shifted from focusing on what wasn't possible to savoring what was. They created a weekly *"intimacy date"* where performance was off the table, but affection and playfulness were front and center. *"It took the pressure away,"* the wife said. *"And that's when desire began to return naturally."*

Action Step: Schedule one *"intimacy date"* per week—no expectations, just presence and touch.

3. Medical Tools Without Shame

For many men, medical support—whether pills, vacuum devices, or injections—can help restore function and confidence. Studies show drugs like sildenafil *(Viagra)* or tadalafil *(Cialis)* help about *60% of men* regain erectile function within *18–24 months* post-surgery.[87] Vacuum devices or rehabilitation programs can further promote blood flow and recovery.

These are not crutches—they're tools. Using them does not mean failure; it means resourcefulness. Urologists and sexual health specialists can guide you through the safest and most effective options.

Action Step: At your next urology visit, ask directly: *"What options are available for penile rehabilitation in my situation?"*

4. Kegel Exercise: Pelvic Health

Strong pelvic floor muscles are not just for bladder control—they directly improve erectile firmness and orgasm intensity. Kegel exercises, done consistently, have been shown to reduce urinary leakage and enhance sexual function after prostate cancer treatment.

Here's the bonus: couples can practice them together. Many partners report feeling more engaged when they both follow the same routine—it turns recovery into a team effort.

Action Step: Try this daily: tighten the pelvic muscles (as if stopping urination midstream), hold for 5 seconds, release. Do 10 reps, 3 times a day. Challenge your partner to join you.

5. Emotional Intimacy First: Connection Before Desire

Emotional intimacy often rebuilds physical intimacy. Eye contact, shared hobbies, gratitude rituals, or even humor during awkward moments can rekindle closeness. A meta-analysis found that couples who maintained strong emotional bonds were more likely to report satisfying sexual relationships—even when physical function was limited.[88]

One couple I met laughed about their early struggles with devices, choosing humor over frustration. *"We turned it into a comedy act,"* the husband joked. *"And somehow, that made us closer."*

Action Step: Share one gratitude with your partner every night before bed. It rewires focus away from what cancer took and toward what love still gives.

Remember
Intimacy after cancer is not about *"going back"*—it's about building forward, together.

Three Ways to Give Back

Thriving beyond prostate cancer isn't just about what you do for yourself—it's also about what you contribute to others. Survivorship can sometimes feel like standing on the far shore of a stormy sea, watching others struggle to cross. Giving back allows you to throw out a lifeline, and in doing so, you strengthen your own recovery. Research indicates that survivors who participate in community support, advocacy, or mentorship often report a higher quality of life, lower anxiety levels, and a stronger sense of purpose.

Here are three powerful and practical ways to turn your experience into a legacy of hope.

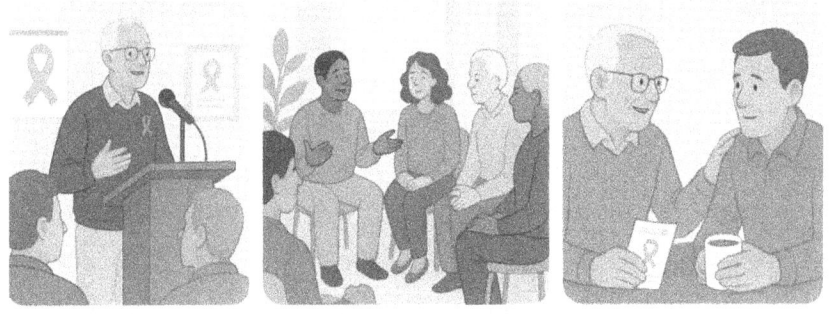

1. Mentorship: Walking Beside the Newly Diagnosed

Hearing the words *"you have prostate cancer"* is overwhelming. Most men don't know what to expect, what questions to ask, or how to cope with the sudden changes. This is where mentorship makes a difference. Survivors who step up as mentors offer more than just advice—they provide perspective, encouragement, and a living example of resilience. Data shows that peer support programs, such as the *Acti-Pair initiative*, help men increase physical activity and motivation during recovery.[89]

It doesn't have to be formal. Sometimes it's a coffee chat, a phone call, or a message exchange. A newly diagnosed man might want to know how you handled PSA anxiety, or what helped you talk openly with your partner about intimacy. Your lived experience is a guidebook no doctor can write.

Action Step: Volunteer for one call, coffee meeting, or group session each month. Even a single conversation can shift someone's outlook from fear to hope.

2. Advocacy: Turning Your Voice into Impact

Sharing your story publicly—whether in a church group, on social media, or at a local health fair—can normalize conversations about prostate cancer and encourage men to seek screening early. Studies show that advocacy work not only helps the community but also improves emotional well-being for survivors, reducing feelings of shame and isolation.

One survivor I worked with began writing short posts on Facebook about his journey with prostate cancer. Within months, several friends told him they had scheduled screenings because of his words. *"If I helped even one person catch this earlier,"* he said, *"then my story has purpose."*

Action Step: Say yes to one opportunity this season—whether speaking at a local event, joining a fundraiser walk, or simply sharing your story online.

3. Support Groups: Finding Strength in Shared Stories

Healing is not a solo act. One of the most powerful ways to give back—and to stay strong—is by joining or helping to lead a support group. These circles provide a safe place to share fears, side effects, and victories with men who truly understand what you're going through. Research shows that prostate cancer survivors who take part in peer groups often report lower distress, improved coping, and even better adherence to treatment plans.

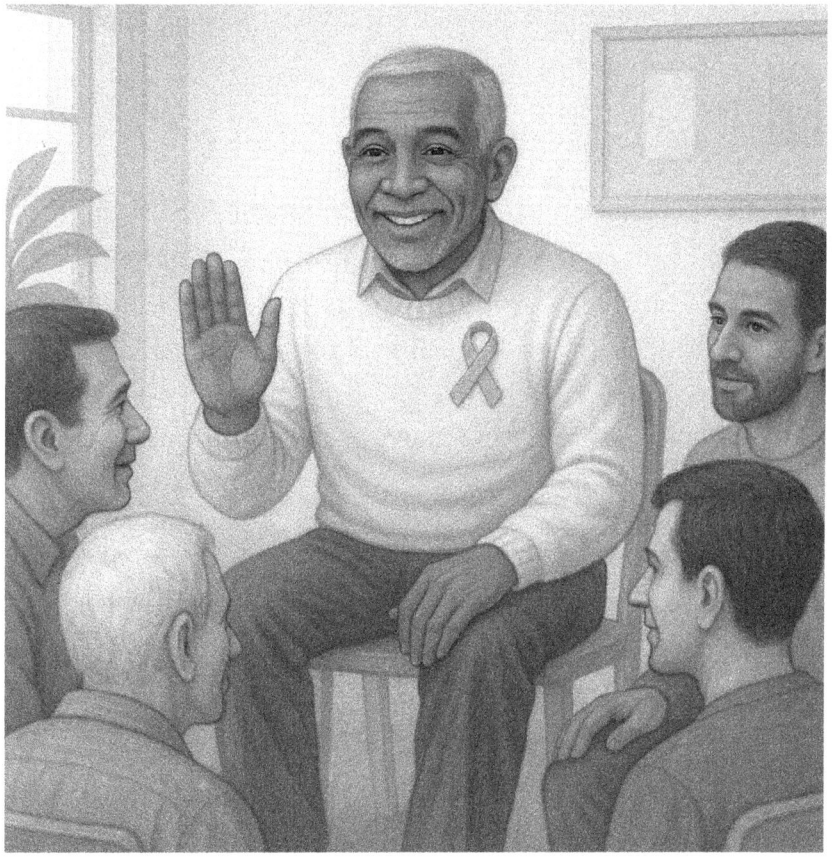

Support groups come in many forms: in-person meetings at hospitals or community centers, or online forums where you can connect with men worldwide. You might simply show up and listen at first, but over time, your story could become the encouragement someone else desperately needs.

I recall one survivor who joined a small local group reluctantly, thinking it "wasn't for him." Months later, he admitted, *"This room became the one place I didn't have to pretend everything was fine. I walked in heavy and walked out lighter."*

Action Step: Commit to attending one support group session—local or virtual—this month. If none exist nearby, consider starting one, even if it begins with just two- or three-men sharing coffee and conversation.

Case Study – Living Beyond Survival

Tom, a 66-year-old veteran, thought the most challenging part was behind him after his prostatectomy in 2020. The surgery was successful, and his PSA dropped to undetectable levels. But the months that followed brought new challenges: erectile dysfunction, bouts of depression, and a constant fear that the cancer might return. *"I felt like I'd lost my purpose,"* he admitted.

At first, Tom retreated into himself, skipping social events and avoiding conversations about his health. But over time, he realized that surviving wasn't enough—he wanted to reclaim his life. His turnaround began with one slight shift: *reframing his mindset*. Each night, he wrote down a single *"victory"* in a journal—whether it was eating a broccoli stir-fry, walking 30 minutes with his dog, or practicing a 10-minute meditation. Those little wins stacked up, reshaping his outlook from victim to victor.

Quarterly PSA monitoring reassured him that his cancer remained under control, staying undetectable (<0.1 ng/mL). At the same time, Tom and his wife sought counseling to address intimacy struggles. Through honest conversations, gentle touch, and patience, they rebuilt closeness that went far beyond performance. *"We learned intimacy is about connection, not just sex,"* he reflected.

Perhaps the biggest transformation came when Tom joined a local prostate cancer support group. At first, he simply listened, but soon he was sharing his own journey. Later, he began volunteering at his VA hospital, mentoring newly diagnosed men and speaking at awareness events. *"Advocacy gave me a mission,"* he said. *"Helping others made me stronger, too."*

Eighteen months later, Tom's PSA remained undetectable, his relationship deepened, and he described feeling more purposeful than at any point in his retirement. His story is echoed in research: a study in the *Journal of Clinical Oncology* found that survivors who engaged in regular vigorous activity had up to a **60% lower risk of prostate cancer death** compared to their sedentary peers.[90] Tom's walking routine, combined with mindfulness and mentoring, wasn't just therapy—it was life extension.

Tom's journey highlights an important truth: thriving after prostate cancer isn't about erasing the past; it's about using it as fuel. By combining mindset shifts, rebuilding intimacy, and giving back, he transformed survivorship into a richer, more connected life.

Key Takeaways

- **Mindset is the foundation.** Shifting from fear to focus, from isolation to connection, and from loss to purpose allows survivors to reclaim their agency and live with intention.

- **Intimacy can be redefined.** Open communication, non-sexual closeness, medical support, and patience help couples rediscover connection and rebuild confidence.

- **Giving back multiplies healing.** Advocacy, mentorship, and survivor networks transform personal struggle into communal strength, creating a purpose that extends beyond survivorship.

- **Habits sustain resilience.** Small daily wins—whether journaling, walking, or practicing meditation—stack up to build long-term vitality.

- **Partnership matters.** Caregivers, spouses, and peers provide the emotional anchors and accountability that make thriving possible.

- **Thriving is a choice.** It's not about perfection but about consistent, intentional actions that transform survivorship into a richer, more meaningful life.

CONCLUSION
DESIGNING YOUR PROSTATE HEALTH FUTURE

You've walked a long road through these pages—from understanding your diagnosis to navigating treatments, exploring alternative therapies, resetting your habits, and learning how to thrive beyond cancer. Along the way, you've seen that prostate cancer is not just a medical condition; it's a life condition. It reshapes how you eat, move, rest, love, and connect. But it does not define you.

If there's one truth this book carries, it's this: **you are not powerless.** Every choice—what's on your plate, how you handle stress, whether you walk or sit, whether you are isolated or connected—nudges your health in a direction. Science is clear: lifestyle shifts can reduce recurrence risk by up to 30%, and complementary approaches can amplify recovery without replacing medical care. Survivorship is not about waiting for the next PSA test; it's about living with intention every single day.

This book has given you:

- **Clarity** on medical treatments and when to say yes—or no—to interventions.
- **Confidence** in daily habits that lower inflammation and strengthen immunity.

- **Tools** for mind-body healing—meditation, yoga, breathwork, and stress resets.
- **A 90-Day Reset** to build momentum with structure, not overwhelm.
- **A Longevity Protocol** to keep cancer at bay and health at the center.
- **A Thriving Blueprint** to rediscover intimacy, connection, and purpose.

Together, these steps form not just a survival plan, but a life plan.

Don't put this book down and let it gather dust. Start today. Pick one action—drink green tea, journal a win, go for a walk, or schedule your PSA. Small, consistent steps create compounding results. Share what you've learned with your partner, your sons, your brothers, or your community. By protecting yourself, you also protect them.

You are more than patient. You are a builder of habits, a connector of families, a source of resilience. Cancer may have started this chapter, but you get to write the ending.

Live your reset. Track your health. Thrive beyond survival.

Your future is not just about years added to your life—it's about life added to your years.

Now it's your turn. Take one action today. Because the best time to reclaim your health, your purpose, and your future is now.

ABOUT THE AUTHOR

Dr. Farhan Mehmood is a physician with over five years of experience treating cancer patients across Pakistan and the United Kingdom. His clinical work spans from rural health centers to modern oncology hospitals—giving him a rare perspective on what patients truly need: not just treatment, but clarity, dignity, and a voice in their care.

His passion for prostate cancer is deeply personal. After witnessing his grandfather's painful battle with the disease—and the silence surrounding it—Dr. Mehmood made a promise: to help men and their families face prostate cancer with knowledge, confidence, and hope.

Trained in conventional oncology and now pursuing advanced studies in integrative medicine, Dr. Mehmood bridges the best of both worlds: science-backed treatments, evidence-based nutrition, and practical mindset tools. His unique 3-Pillar Protocol is built to empower—not overwhelm—patients at every stage of their journey.

When he's not working with patients or writing health guides, Dr. Mehmood mentors young doctors from underserved communities and speaks out for accessible, compassionate cancer care worldwide.

REFERENCES

1. Prostate Cancer Survival Rates. https://www.webmd.com/prostate-cancer/prostate-cancer-survival-rates-what-they-mean.

2. Chu, F. *et al.* Global burden of prostate cancer: age-period-cohort analysis from 1990 to 2021 and projections until 2040. *World J Surg Oncol* 23, 98 (2025).

3. Key Statistics for Prostate Cancer | Prostate Cancer Facts | American Cancer Society. https://www.cancer.org/cancer/types/prostate-cancer/about/key-statistics.html.

4. Siegel, R. L., Kratzer, T. B., Giaquinto, A. N., Sung, H. & Jemal, A. Cancer statistics, 2025. *CA Cancer J Clin* 75, 10–45 (2025).

5. Jain, M. A., Leslie, S. W. & Sapra, A. Prostate Cancer Screening. *StatPearls* https://www.ncbi.nlm.nih.gov/books/NBK556081/ (2023).

6. Mccaffery, K. *et al.* Resisting recommended treatment for prostate cancer: a qualitative analysis of the lived experience of possible overdiagnosis. *BMJ Open* 9, e026960 (2019).

7. Gore, A. Needle Biopsy market size will be USD 1.71 Billion by 2030! https://www.cognitivemarketresearch.com/needle-biopsy-market-report (2025).

8. McConnell, J. D. *et al.* The Long-Term Effect of Doxazosin, Finasteride, and Combination Therapy on the Clinical

Progression of Benign Prostatic Hyperplasia. *New England Journal of Medicine* 349, 2387–2398 (2003).

9. Madhushankha, M., Jayarajah, U. & Abeygunasekera, A. M. Clinical characteristics, etiology, management and outcome of hematospermia: a systematic review. *Am J Clin Exp Urol* 9, 1 (2021).

10. Smith, A. E., Muralidharan, A. & Smith, M. T. Prostate cancer induced bone pain: pathobiology, current treatments and pain responses from recent clinical trials. *Discover. Oncology* 13, 108 (2022).

11. Kinnaird, W. *et al.* Sexual Dysfunction in Prostate Cancer Patients According to Disease Stage and Treatment Modality. *Clin Oncol* 41, 103801 (2025).

12. Smith, D. T., Mouzon, D. M. & Elliott, M. Reviewing the Assumptions About Men's Mental Health: An Exploration of the Gender Binary. *Am J Mens Health* 12, 78 (2016).

13. Sharma, M. & Miyamoto, H. Percent Gleason pattern 4 in stratifying the prognosis of patients with intermediate-risk prostate cancer. *Transl Androl Urol* 7, S484 (2018).

14. Breyer, B. N. *et al.* Updates to Incontinence After Prostate Treatment: AUA/GURS/SUFU Guideline (2024). *Journal of Urology* 212, 531–538 (2024).

15. Monda, S. M. *et al.* Trends in Surgical Overtreatment of Prostate Cancer. *JAMA Oncol* https://doi.org/10.1001/JAMAONCOL.2025.0963 (2025) doi:10.1001/JAMAONCOL.2025.0963.

16. Egevad, L. *et al.* Prognosis of Gleason Score 9–10 Prostatic Adenocarcinoma in Needle Biopsies: A Nationwide Population-based Study. *Eur Urol Oncol* 7, 213–221 (2024).

17. Allan, C. A., Collins, V. R., Frydenberg, M., Mclachlan, R. I. & Matthiesson, K. L. Monitoring cardiovascular health in men with prostate cancer treated with androgen deprivation therapy. *International Journal of Urological Nursing* 6, 35–41 (2012).

18. Myint, Z. W. & Kunos, C. A. Bone Fracture Incidence After Androgen Deprivation Therapy-Investigational Agents: Results From Cancer Therapy Evaluation Program-Sponsored Early Phase Clinical Trials 2006–2013. *Front Oncol* 10, 1125 (2020).

19. Flores, I. E. *et al.* Stress alters the expression of cancer-related genes in the prostate. *BMC Cancer* 17, 1–10 (2017).

20. BRCA Genes & Prostate Cancer | PCFA. https://www.prostate.org.au/testing-and-diagnosis/grading-genetics/genetic-risks-testing/brca-genes-prostate-cancer/.

21. Foerster, B. *et al.* Association of Smoking Status With Recurrence, Metastasis, and Mortality Among Patients With Localized Prostate Cancer Undergoing Prostatectomy or Radiotherapy: A Systematic Review and Meta-analysis. *JAMA Oncol* 4, 953–961 (2018).

22. Woloshin, S. *et al.* Updating the Know Your Chances Website to Include Smoking Status as a Risk Factor for Mortality Estimates. *JAMA Netw Open* 6, e2317351–e2317351 (2023).

23. Key Statistics for Prostate Cancer | Prostate Cancer Facts | American Cancer Society. https://www.cancer.org/cancer/types/prostate-cancer/about/key-statistics.html.

24. Prostate Cancer — Cancer Stat Facts. https://seer.cancer.gov/statfacts/html/prost.html.

25. Prostate-Specific Antigen (PSA) Test - NCI. https://www.cancer.gov/types/prostate/psa-fact-sheet.

26. Lumbreras, B. *et al.* Variables Associated with False-Positive PSA Results: A Cohort Study with Real-World Data. *Cancers 2023, Vol. 15, Page 261* 15, 261 (2022).

27. Thompson, I. M. *et al.* Prevalence of Prostate Cancer among Men with a Prostate-Specific Antigen Level ≤4.0 ng per Milliliter. *New England Journal of Medicine* 350, 2239–2246 (2004).

28. Tchetgen, M. B., Song, J. T., Strawderman, M., Jacobsen, S. J. & Oesterling, J. E. Ejaculation increases the serum prostate-specific antigen concentration. *Urology* 47, 511–516 (1996).

29. Chybowski, F. M., Bergstralh, E. J. & Oesterling, J. E. The effect of digital rectal examination on the serum prostate specific antigen concentration: results of a randomized study. *J Urol* 148, 83–86 (1992).

30. Loeb, S., Roehl, K. A., Catalona, W. J. & Nadler, R. B. Prostate specific antigen velocity threshold for predicting prostate cancer in young men. *J Urol* 177, 899–902 (2007).

31. EAU Guidelines - Uroweb. https://uroweb.org/guidelines.

32. Fletcher, P. *et al.* Vector Prostate Biopsy: A Novel Magnetic Resonance Imaging/Ultrasound Image Fusion Transperineal Biopsy Technique Using Electromagnetic Needle Tracking Under Local Anaesthesia. *Eur Urol* 83, 249–256 (2023).

33. Wenzel, M. *et al.* Complication Rates After TRUS Guided Transrectal Systematic and MRI-Targeted Prostate Biopsies in a High-Risk Region for Antibiotic Resistances. *Front Surg* 7, 7 (2020).

34. Wang, N. N. *et al.* Applying the PRECISION approach in biopsy naïve and previously negative prostate biopsy patients.

Urologic Oncology: Seminars and Original Investigations 37, 530.e19-530.e24 (2019).

35. Prices for Transrectal ultrasound services | Turquoise Health. https://turquoise.health/services/transrectal-ultrasound/.

36. Prostate Biopsy: Pros and Cons. https://www.news-medical.net/health/Prostate-Biopsy-Pros-and-Cons.aspx.

37. Vakili, S. *et al.* Transforming Prostate Cancer Care: Innovations in Diagnosis, Treatment, and Future Directions. *International Journal of Molecular Sciences 2025, Vol. 26, Page 5386* 26, 5386 (2025).

38. Kang, H. C. *et al.* Accuracy of Prostate Magnetic Resonance Imaging: Reader Experience Matters. *Eur Urol Open Sci* 27, 53–60 (2021).

39. Okubo, Y. *et al.* Diagnostic significance of reassessment of prostate biopsy specimens by experienced urological pathologists at a high-volume institution. *Virchows Archiv* 480, 979–987 (2022).

40. Zhang, Y. *et al.* A comprehensive analysis of erectile dysfunction prevalence and the impact of prostate conditions on ED among US adults: evidence from NHANES 2001-2004. *Front Endocrinol (Lausanne)* 15, 1412369 (2024).

41. Wu, S. Y., Chang, C. L., Chen, C. I. & Huang, C. C. Comparison of Acute and Chronic Surgical Complications Following Robot-Assisted, Laparoscopic, and Traditional Open Radical Prostatectomy Among Men in Taiwan. *JAMA Netw Open* 4, e2120156–e2120156 (2021).

42. Capogrosso, P., Salonia, A., Briganti, A. & Montorsi, F. Postprostatectomy Erectile Dysfunction: A Review. *World J Mens Health* 34, 73–88 (2016).

43. Urinary Dysfunction After Prostate Cancer Treatment | Johns Hopkins Medicine. https://www.hopkinsmedicine.org/health/treatment-tests-and-therapies/urinary-dysfunction-after-prostate-cancer-treatment.

44. Tatenuma, T. *et al.* Association of hospital volume with perioperative and oncological outcomes of robot-assisted laparoscopic radical prostatectomy: a retrospective multicenter cohort study. *BMC Urol* 23, 1–7 (2023).

45. Bowel Dysfunction After Prostate Cancer Treatment | Johns Hopkins Medicine. https://www.hopkinsmedicine.org/health/treatment-tests-and-therapies/bowel-dysfunction-after-prostate-cancer-treatment.

46. SBRT Proves Effective for Some Prostate Cancers - NCI. https://www.cancer.gov/news-events/cancer-currents-blog/2024/prostate-cancer-sbrt-effective-safe.

47. Pan, H. Y. *et al.* Comparative Toxicities and Cost of Intensity-Modulated Radiotherapy, Proton Radiation, and Stereotactic Body Radiotherapy Among Younger Men With Prostate Cancer. *Journal of Clinical Oncology* 36, 1823–1830 (2018).

48. Proton Therapy For Cancer | American Cancer Society. https://www.cancer.org/cancer/managing-cancer/treatment-types/radiation/proton-therapy.html.

49. The cost-value argument for expanding proton therapy coverage – National Association for Proton Therapy. https://proton-therapy.org/the-cost-value-argument-for-expanding-proton-therapy-coverage/.

50. Proton Therapy for Prostate Cancer | The UF Health Proton Therapy Institute.

https://www.floridaproton.org/ppc/proton-prostate-gainesville.

51. Kantoff, P. W. *et al.* Sipuleucel-T immunotherapy for castration-resistant prostate cancer. *N Engl J Med* 363, 411–422 (2010).

52. Home | ClinicalTrials.gov. https://clinicaltrials.gov/.

53. Crouzet, S. *et al.* Whole-gland ablation of localized prostate cancer with high-intensity focused ultrasound: Oncologic outcomes and morbidity in 1002 patients. *Eur Urol* 65, 907–914 (2014).

54. HIFU Denied By Your Insurance? | Appeal Your Denial Today. https://www.scottglovsky.com/insurance-bad-faith/health-insurance-claim-denials/high-intensity-focused-ultrasound/.

55. Cerbone, L., Regine, G. & Calabrò, F. Active surveillance in low- and intermediate-risk prostate cancer. *Asian J Androl* 26, 582 (2024).

56. Siegel, R. L., Miller, K. D., Wagle, N. S. & Jemal, A. Cancer statistics, 2023. *CA Cancer J Clin* 73, 17–48 (2023).

57. Giovannucci, E., Rimm, E. B., Liu, Y., Stampfer, M. J. & Willett, W. C. A prospective study of tomato products, lycopene, and prostate cancer risk. *J Natl Cancer Inst* 94, 391–398 (2002).

58. Pantuck, A. J. *et al.* Phase II study of pomegranate juice for men with rising prostate-specific antigen following surgery or radiation for prostate cancer. *Clin Cancer Res* 12, 4018–4026 (2006).

59. Kirsh, V. A. *et al.* Prospective study of fruit and vegetable intake and risk of prostate cancer. *J Natl Cancer Inst* 99, 1200–1209 (2007).

60. Kurahashi, N., Sasazuki, S., Iwasaki, M. & Inoue, M. Green tea consumption and prostate cancer risk in Japanese men: a prospective study. *Am J Epidemiol* 167, 71–77 (2008).

61. Szymanski, K. M., Wheeler, D. C. & Mucci, L. A. Fish consumption and prostate cancer risk: A review and meta-analysis. *American Journal of Clinical Nutrition* 92, 1223–1233 (2010).

62. Yan, L. & Spitznagel, E. L. Soy consumption and prostate cancer risk in men: A revisit of a meta-analysis. *American Journal of Clinical Nutrition* 89, 1155–1163 (2009).

63. Wang, W. *et al.* Nut consumption and prostate cancer risk and mortality. *Br J Cancer* 115, 371 (2016).

64. Kunnumakkara, A. B. *et al.* Curcumin mediates anticancer effects by modulating multiple cell signaling pathways. *Clin Sci (Lond)* 131, 1781–1799 (2017).

65. Serenoa repens for benign prostatic hyperplasia - Tacklind, J - 2012 | Cochrane Library. https://www.cochranelibrary.com/cdsr/doi/10.1002/14651858.CD001423.pub3/full.

66. Macoska, J. A. The use of beta-sitosterol for the treatment of prostate cancer and benign prostatic hyperplasia. *Am J Clin Exp Urol* 11, 467 (2023).

67. Victorson, D. *et al.* Mindfulness-Based Stress Reduction for Men on Active Surveillance for Prostate Cancer and their Spouses: Design and Methodology of a Randomized Controlled Trial. *Contemp Clin Trials* 125, 107059 (2022).

68. Kox, M. *et al.* Voluntary activation of the sympathetic nervous system and attenuation of the innate immune response in humans. *Proc Natl Acad Sci U S A* 111, 7379–7384 (2014).

69. Jafari, M. *et al.* Effect of Acupressure on Pain and Sleep Quality of Patients with Cancer after Undergoing Surgery Admitted to

the Intensive Care Unit: A Single-blind Randomized Clinical Trial. *Iran J Nurs Midwifery Res* 30, 531 (2025).

70. Wang, M. *et al.* The role of deep hyperthermia in IMRT in elderly patients with esophageal cancer: a retrospective cohort study. *Radiat Oncol* 20, 76 (2025).

71. Wagle, N. S. *et al.* Cancer treatment and survivorship statistics, 2025. *CA Cancer J Clin* 75, 308–340 (2025).

72. Rabbani, S. A. *et al.* Impact of Lifestyle Modifications on Cancer Mortality: A Systematic Review and Meta-Analysis. *Medicina (Lithuania)* 61, 307 (2025).

73. PDQ Adult Treatment Editorial Board. Prostate Cancer Treatment (PDQ®). *PDQ Cancer Information Summaries* 1–115 (2022).

74. Mottet, N. *et al.* EAU-EANM-ESTRO-ESUR-SIOG Guidelines on Prostate Cancer—2020 Update. Part 1: Screening, Diagnosis, and Local Treatment with Curative Intent. *Eur Urol* 79, 243–262 (2021).

75. Hofman, M. S. *et al.* Prostate-specific membrane antigen PET-CT in patients with high-risk prostate cancer before curative-intent surgery or radiotherapy (proPSMA): a prospective, randomised, multicentre study. *The Lancet* 395, 1208–1216 (2020).

76. Pound, C. R. *et al.* Natural history of progression after PSA elevation following radical prostatectomy. *J Am Med Assoc* 281, 1591–1597 (1999).

77. Healthy Eating - American Institute for Cancer Research. https://www.aicr.org/cancer-prevention/healthy-eating/.

78. Cao, Y. & Ma, J. Body mass index, prostate cancer-specific mortality, and biochemical recurrence: A systematic review

and meta-analysis. *Cancer Prevention Research* 4, 486–501 (2011).

79. Darcey, E. & Boyle, T. Tobacco smoking and survival after a prostate cancer diagnosis: A systematic review and meta-analysis. *Cancer Treat Rev* 70, 30–40 (2018).

80. Markt, S. C. *et al.* Sleep duration and disruption and prostate cancer risk: a 23-year prospective study. *Cancer Epidemiol Biomarkers Prev* 25, 302 (2015).

81. Diaphragmatic Breathing Exercises & Benefits. https://my.clevelandclinic.org/health/articles/9445-diaphragmatic-breathing.

82. Advanced Prostate Cancer. https://www.urotoday.com/library-resources/advanced-prostate-cancer.html.

83. Kenfield, S. A., Stampfer, M. J., Giovannucci, E. & Chan, J. M. Physical activity and survival after prostate cancer diagnosis in the health professionals follow-up study. *J Clin Oncol* 29, 726–732 (2011).

84. Lebel, S. *et al.* From normal response to clinical problem: definition and clinical features of fear of cancer recurrence. *Support Care Cancer* 24, 3265–3268 (2016).

85. Sharp, L., O'Leary, E., Kinnear, H., Gavin, A. & Drummond, F. J. Cancer-related symptoms predict psychological wellbeing among prostate cancer survivors: results from the PiCTure study. *Psychooncology* 25, 282–291 (2016).

86. Fergus, K. *et al.* Couplelinks - an online intervention for young women with breast cancer and their male partners: study protocol for a randomized controlled trial. *Trials* 16, 33 (2015).

87. Matthew, A. G. *et al.* SEXUAL DYSFUNCTION AFTER RADICAL PROSTATECTOMY: PREVALENCE, TREATMENTS,

RESTRICTED USE OF TREATMENTS AND DISTRESS. *J Urol* 174, 2105–2110 (2005).

88. Tal, R., Alphs, H. H., Krebs, P., Nelson, C. J. & Mulhall, J. P. Erectile Function Recovery Rate after Radical Prostatectomy: A Meta-Analysis. *J Sex Med* 6, 2538 (2009).

89. Baudot, A. *et al.* The Acti-Pair program helps men with prostate cancer increase physical activity with peer support: a mixed method pilot study. *Front Public Health* 11, 1321230 (2023).

90. Kenfield, S. A., Stampfer, M. J., Giovannucci, E. & Chan, J. M. Physical Activity and Survival After Prostate Cancer Diagnosis in the Health Professionals Follow-Up Study. *Journal of Clinical Oncology* 29, 726 (2011).

GLOSSARY OF TERMS

ADT (Androgen Deprivation Therapy): A treatment that lowers levels of male hormones (androgens) like testosterone, which fuel prostate cancer growth.

BPH (Benign Prostatic Hyperplasia): A non-cancerous enlargement of the prostate that can cause urinary problems.

BRCA (BRCA1/BRCA2 Genes): Genes that, when mutated, can increase the risk of breast, ovarian, and prostate cancers.

Biopsy: A medical procedure that removes small samples of prostate tissue, usually with a needle, to check for cancer under a microscope.

CTC (Circulating Tumor Cells): Cancer cells that break away from the prostate tumor and circulate in the bloodstream, sometimes used in research to monitor disease.

Erectile Dysfunction: Difficulty achieving or maintaining an erection, often caused by prostate cancer or its treatments.

Gleason Score: A grading system that describes how abnormal prostate cancer cells look under a microscope. Scores range from 6 to 10, with higher numbers indicating a more aggressive cancer.

HIFU (High-Intensity Focused Ultrasound): A treatment that uses focused sound waves to heat and destroy prostate cancer cells while sparing surrounding tissue.

Hyperthermia: A therapy that uses heat to make cancer cells more sensitive to radiation or chemotherapy.

IMRT (Intensity-Modulated Radiation Therapy): A precise form of external radiation that shapes beams to the prostate, reducing damage to nearby organs.

Immunotherapy: A treatment that helps the body's immune system recognize and attack prostate cancer cells.

Incontinence: Loss of bladder control, which may occur after prostate surgery or radiation.

MRI (Magnetic Resonance Imaging): An imaging test that uses magnets and radio waves to create detailed pictures of the prostate and surrounding tissues.

Nocturia: Frequent urination at night, which may be linked to prostate problems.

Oncology: The branch of medicine that deals with the study and treatment of cancer.

PET Scan (Positron Emission Tomography): An imaging test that uses a radioactive tracer to detect cancer spread. PSMA PET scans are especially sensitive for prostate cancer.

PSA (Prostate-Specific Antigen): A protein made by the prostate. PSA levels are measured through blood tests and used to screen for and monitor prostate cancer.

PSA Velocity: The rate at which PSA levels rise over time. A faster increase may suggest prostate cancer progression or recurrence.

Proton Therapy: A type of radiation that uses protons instead of X-rays, reducing exposure to nearby healthy tissues.

Radiation Therapy: A treatment that uses high-energy beams to kill prostate cancer cells while sparing nearby healthy tissue.

Robotic Surgery: A minimally invasive surgical technique for removing the prostate using robotic instruments for greater precision.

SBRT (Stereotactic Body Radiation Therapy): A type of radiation therapy that delivers high doses in a small number of sessions with high accuracy.

Ultrasound: An imaging technique that uses sound waves to create pictures of the prostate. Often used to guide biopsies.

www.ingramcontent.com/pod-product-compliance
Lightning Source LLC
Chambersburg PA
CBHW051549020426
42333CB00016B/2172